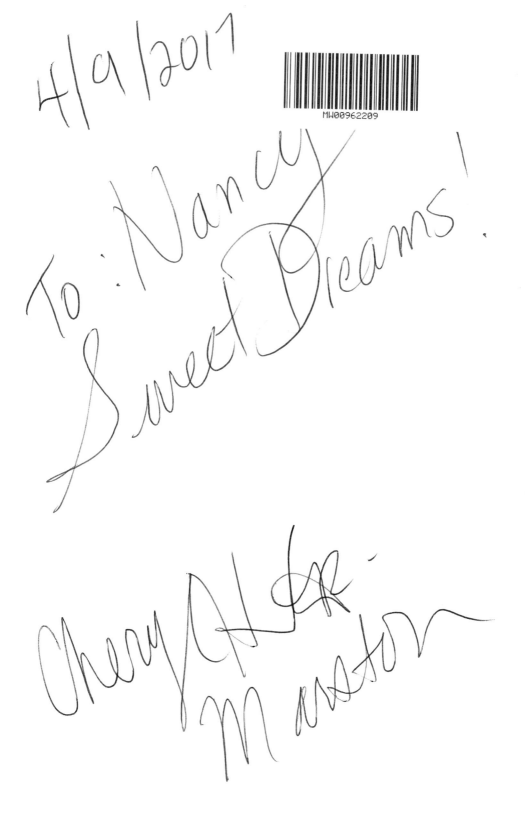

4/9/2017

To : Nancy

Sweet Dreams !

Cheryl

Manston

SLEEP
is
GOD'S
MEDICINE

Understanding and Appreciating
His Therapeutic Gift of Sleep

CHERYL HUNTER-MARSTON

WESTBOW
PRESS®
A DIVISION OF THOMAS NELSON
& ZONDERVAN

WestBow Press books may be ordered through booksellers or by contacting:

WestBow Press
A Division of Thomas Nelson & Zondervan
1663 Liberty Drive
Bloomington, IN 47403
www.westbowpress.com
1 (866) 928-1240

ISBN: 978-1-5127-4880-2 (sc)
ISBN: 978-1-5127-4881-9 (hc)
ISBN: 978-1-5127-4879-6 (e)

Library of Congress Control Number: 2016947255

Print information available on the last page.

WestBow Press rev. date: 10/12/2016

Disclaimer:

The information in this book is not meant to imply that if you have a sleep disorder, there is something wrong with your relationship with God or that you have done something wrong. In this life illness and adversity are part of the human condition. Understanding this, if you have a sleep disorder, there are things in your life that you can modify to help improve your lot in life: manage your stress, pay attention to your diet and other aspects of your daily nutrition, exercise regularly, and if you need to, lose some weight.

Please do not neglect to seek proper professional medical advice for any problems you or your family might notice that interfere with sleeping. Sleep disorders and other sleep-related medical conditions are evaluated by sleep studies ordered by your health-care professional. If you believe you have a sleep disorder, you should seek the advice of a health-care professional regarding your particular medical condition. Detrimental life-altering changes related to chronic sleep deprivation or sleep disorders sometimes can be quite insidious, and thus it is very difficult to ascertain and attribute their cause.

In addition, the information provided in this book is for personal, noncommercial, and educational purposes only and does not constitute a recommendation or endorsement with respect to any company, product, or service. The author makes no representations and specifically disclaims all warranties, express, implied, or statutory, regarding the accuracy, timeliness, completeness, merchantability, or fitness for any particular purpose of any material contained in this book. Information contained in this book is not a substitute for seeking appropriate medical attention.

Unless otherwise indicated, all biblical quotations are from the New International Version® of the Bible.

CONTENTS

Preface viii

Acknowledgments xiv

1   Sleep in the Bible 1
     The Big Sleep 5
     Why Has God Made Sleep Necessary? 8

2   Medicine in the Bible 11

3   Theories of Sleep 14
     Sleep Theories from Classical Antiquity 14
     Early Industrial Age Sleep Theory: Fetal
     Regression, 1856–1939 17
     Modern Schools of Thought 17

4   Anthropology of Sleep 19

5   Sleep Architecture (Sleep Patterns) and Physiology 23

6   Sleep Loss, Sleep Deprivation, and Sleep Debt 33
     Consequences of Long-Term Sleep Loss 34
     Sleep Loss in the Hospitalized Patient 51

7   Holistic Benefits of Sleep 57
     Why Do We Dream When We Sleep? 60

8   Principles of Good Sleep Hygiene or Sleep
     Premedication 68

9   Complementary and Alternative Therapies for a
Good Night's Sleep 87
        Supplement CAT 88
        Other, Non-Supplement CAT 91
        Foods that Promote Sleep 98

10   A Hard Day's Night: How Do Shift Workers Manage?... 100

11   Sleep Throughout the Life Cycle 107
        Sleep in the Newborn and Young Infancy 107
        Sleep In the Toddler Age 111
        Sleep in School-Age Children 113
        Sleep in Adolescence 116
        Sleep During the College Years 124
        Sleep in Adult Women – A Look at
            Pregnancy and Menopause 128
        Sleep in Adult Men 142
        Sleep in Older Adults... 144

12   Count Your Many Blessings, Not Sheep...................... 148

Afterword.. 151
        Sleep Health History Example............................ 160
        Sleep Diary Example 165

Resources 175
        Sleep-Friendly Websites 175
        Sleep Disorder Centers in the United States...... 176

Bibliography.. 179

PREFACE

God created our need for sleep, yet sleep is rarely the theme of any literary writings or the primary topic of discussion in the Bible. It is most often covered as a small part of a larger discussion or exposé on other topics. It is important to see regular sleep as it is—a gift from God. It is His miraculous therapeutic gift.

"For since the creation of the world His invisible attributes are clearly seen, being understood by the things that are made, even His eternal power and Godhead" (Rom. 1:20).

For the scientist and health-care professional, this book is a much lighter review of a small portion of the scientific knowledge regarding sleep. It is Sleep 101 from another perspective. In this book one will find many references to Scripture because, although the Bible is not a medical science text, it speaks of medical science with divine insight and accuracy.

"That which has been is what will be,
That which is done is what will be done,
And there is nothing new under the sun" (Eccl. 1:9).

God created science to help us understand and discover the wonders of His world. For Him in regard to all knowledge, nothing is new. Therefore, we must not beat ourselves up because our state-of-the-art scientific research is just our current best-educated guess in unlocking all the secrets and mystery of sleep science. God did not intend that knowledge about health and healing be solely the domain of the health care provider. By establishing a mutual sharing relationship between caregiver and patient, untold benefits can be gained on the road to achieving great health and well-being. It is fitting that health-care providers understand and let their patients know that in obtaining an optimum amount of sleep each night, they are cooperating with God in the work of restoration and recuperation.

Many of us unduly suffer due to the detrimental practice of intentionally not getting the proper rest and sleep that we need in order to maintain good health and well-being. God created sleep for the benefit of our physical bodies and our spiritual and mental well-being. In this sense, sleep is God's medicine. God did not intend for the spiritual life to be separate from the physical—holistically they are one! Acknowledging and understanding this fact is crucial for those who are called and committed to the ministry of healing.

For the layperson, this book is a not-too-technical review of sleep and sleep science. My hope is that everyone will gain some very interesting insights into the essential phenomenon of sleep and the miracle of sleep as God's medicine.

Although this book is primarily for adult men and women, hopefully it will also inspire adults to use the information contained herein to promote healthier lifestyles for our grade school-age children and teens, who continue to reap serious negative consequences from lack of sleep.

Still, one might ask the question, why write a book entitled *Sleep Is God's Medicine*? In reality, many people already have a good working knowledge of the lifestyle changes and sleep habits that they should adopt in order to avail themselves of more restful and therapeutic sleep. However, often with self-management health programs or health and wellness therapies, there remains a significant amount of complacency and noncompliance. Why is this? Because for many there is no deep emotional or spiritual commitment to long-lasting change or adherence to prescribed or recommended therapeutic interventions.

It is my hope that through a clear, deep understanding and appreciation of *Sleep Is God's Medicine*, many individuals will be inspired to make the necessary lifestyle changes and appropriate therapeutic interventions sufficient to obtain better sleep. Making these changes permanent, I believe, will result in not only a significant difference in the reader's overall quality of life but will also help readers along this life's earthly and spiritual journey.

I have a history of insomnia, and on occasion I still suffer from it. Despite this occasional problem, I often dream very vivid, lucid dreams. According to the Lucidity Institute Inc., founded in 1987 by Stephen LaBerge, "lucid dreaming" means "dreaming while knowing you are dreaming" and consciously guiding the direction of your dreams LaBerge (2007). He suggested that becoming aware of lucid dreaming could help people become more creative and better able to solve problems. This has certainly been true for me. Many creative revelations and ideas have come to me while in deep sleep, including the spiritual encouragement to write this book.

Many years ago while a young college student at Stanford University, I took the immensely popular Sleep and Dreams course taught by William C. Dement, MD (now professor emeritus, and who by most expert opinions is still considered to be the father of modern sleep medicine and research). This experience started me on a lifelong fascination with sleep. For many years I pondered the question, "Why does God have us spend approximately one third of our precious time here on earth sleeping?" Hopefully after reading this book, the reader will come to realize that we truly need the approximate eight-hour infusion of sleep in order to participate in all the miraculous therapeutic and restorative activities that occur during sleep. In other words readers will come to understand and value that sleep is God's medicine.

In humble recognition and acceptance of His plan for our lives, we should do all things to His glory and honor (most importantly building the kingdom of God). Every day we must rely on the Holy Spirit working in us and through us to accomplish His will. We will not able to work out our salvation through our own physical strength or by our own human effort, yet we still need our physical strength to accomplish these things.

Now you may still be asking yourself the question: "Why is it so important that we come to the realization that sleep is God's medicine?" The Scriptures state that every good and perfect gift comes from God above. Thus, we should be thankful and appreciative of sleep, this miraculous therapeutic gift of God.

"For so He gives his beloved sleep" (Ps. 127:2).

In our 24-7 society, many have adopted the cultural mindset that it is completely acceptable to neglect our sleep. There is a highly visible love affair between lightning-speed mobile communication and the high-pressure demand for twenty-four-hour accessibility to goods and services. In our fast-paced contemporary society, we receive many signals that help us rationalize this love affair—pressures to be more, to do more, and even to say more. Yet we should stop and ask ourselves what we are really missing that is so vitally important when we pause from the day's activities to devote eight hours a night to sleeping—that late-night movie, reality TV reruns, the shopping channel or infomercial, or some late-night partying? Oh, yes, let's not forget the wonderful opportunity to go sightseeing by the light of the silvery moon!

Unfortunately, too many people view dedicating eight hours of the day to sleep as an irresponsible activity. It is as if we relish the idea of proving how busy and important our lives are by wearing our resultant sleep deprivation as some sort of badge of sacrifice and honor. This widespread practice of burning the candle at both ends, as previously stated, is often a sign of disproportionate desire to do more, accomplish more, or function within our own power, not in God's power and will.

"This is the word of the LORD to Zerubbabel: 'Not by might nor by power, but by my Spirit,' says the LORD Almighty" (Zech. 4:6).

For many of us, regular skipping on sleep has become the norm or routine. Many of us have fallen into the trap of marginalizing our sleep needs through a catch-22 scenario. We give in to pressures and perceived requirements to be more productive or efficient and ignore our sleep; then over time we become chronically sleep-deprived. As a result, we begin to feel that we are not as productive or efficient in what we must or should be doing in the daytime (which is true because we are sleep-deprived!), and then this vicious cycle just keeps repeating.

During the course of writing this book, it was very important for me not to fall prey to this unhealthy habit. I had to emotionally learn what sleep researchers have told us for years: that one must not confuse being awake with wakefulness. As with rest and relaxation, sleep serves the purpose of preparing one for labor and other energy-consuming activities. Lost shut-eye or sleep-related problems are the prime reasons many people call in sick or come in late to work.

During sleep, miraculous events of restoration, rejuvenation, and growth occur, which no drug will ever come close to replicating in form or function. Therefore, we now know that *Sleep Is God's Medicine.*

ACKNOWLEDGMENTS

First, thanks and praise go to God our Father. Were it not for His persistent nudging, inspiration, and guidance, this book would not have been written. My appreciation is extended to two sleep disorder centers, the Stanford Sleep Disorders Center for giving me an extensive tour of their facilities and a review of their services and also the Mercy San Juan Sleep Center for a tour of their facility and the opportunity to observe a sleep study.

I am also deeply indebted to the generosity and loving kindness of mentors Rev. Milton Woods, MD, and the late Rev. Elliott J. "Dad" Mason, Sr., PhD, for their spiritual guidance, prayers, and medical advice in completing this book. Heartfelt thanks are given to other physician friends who shared with me "hallway" advice and additional information on the various medical specialties touched upon in this book. The friends who gave me their loving support and critique along the road to publishing—to them I say thank you, too.

A special thank you is given to my sister-in-law Charis Marston Cardeno, PhD, and the Grand Canyon University Reference Librarians who were instrumental in helping me conduct background article research for *Sleep Is God's Medicine*. A world of gratitude and thanks go to my dearly departed "Aunt Doll" and my sister Melanie D. Hunter, MD. I will never be able to express in words my feelings of love and gratitude for my most beloved mother and best friend, Erma D. Hunter, whose unconditional love always sustained me, and even though she has left us to be with God, continues to sustain me.

Finally, my deepest love and appreciation go to my other best friend, my husband, Kirk M. Marston. Were it not for his unwavering loyal support in difficult times, it would have been very difficult to have made it through to the completion of this book. Much appreciation and thanks go to him for enduring so many disturbances in his life and routine during the writing of this book. His support in so many ways has been priceless.

CHAPTER 1

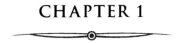

Sleep in the Bible

In the Bible the most common Greek noun for literal sleep is *hupnos* (from which we adopt our English word *hypnosis*), and the Hebrew word is *shenah*. The Greek verb is *katheudo*, and the Hebrew verb is *shakhabh*. *Webster's Universal College Dictionary* defines sleep as "the rest afforded by a suspension of voluntary bodily functions and the natural suspension, complete or partial, of consciousness."

In the Old Testament, deep sleep comes from a root word meaning "to be deaf" (the Hebrew noun is *tardemah*, and the verb is *radham*). The following passages speak to deep sleep:

> So David took the spear and the water jug near Saul's head, and they left. No one saw or knew about it, nor did anyone wake up. They were all sleeping, because the Lord had put them in a deep sleep. (1 Sam. 26:12)

> But Jonah had gone below deck where he lay down and fell into a deep sleep. (Jonah 1:5)

Sleep is also referred to symbolically and figuratively in the Bible. Later in this book, there will be a short description of one of these figurative meanings of sleep as death.

Biblical tradition maintains that at the very creation of the earth, which was followed closely by the separation of the light from darkness, God created rhythms to control the earth: "God called the light 'Day,' and the darkness He called 'Night.' And there was evening and there was morning, the first day" (Gen. 1:5). He required the rhythm of light and darkness to exist before the plants, animals, and even before humans could exist and survive. It is this circadian rhythm (circadian is Latin for "around a day") that informs our bodies when to secrete hormones and when it is time to sleep.

Circadian sleep rhythms are regular changes in sleep characteristics that occur in the course of a day. When the time comes, the human body displays a drive to sleep. When this drive is relieved by an adequate night's sleep, this, along with the body's internal clock, regulates awakening in the morning, unless one has a sleep disorder. This circadian rhythm results in a diurnal variation in the sleep drive, producing two peaks: one between 2:00 a.m. and 4:00 a.m. and a second between 1:00 p.m. and 3:00 p.m. It is this second period that makes most of us sleepy in the early afternoon, not a heavy lunch as we have been taught to think. The circadian rhythm is controlled by what we call the body's biological clock. A regular morning waking time strengthens our circadian rhythm's functioning and helps with sleep onset at night. This is the reason it is so important to keep a regular bedtime and arise and shine to God's glory at a regular wake time, even on the weekends, when sometimes the temptation to sleep in is so great.

As we progress through the biblical story, we understand that God created sleep; yes, the miracle of sleep is the result of divine intervention: "And the LORD God caused a deep sleep to fall on Adam, and he slept; and He took one of his ribs, and closed up the flesh in its place. Then the rib which the LORD God had taken from man He made into a woman" (Gen. 2:21–22). In this sense, God used sleep as a general anesthesia when performing the first transplant surgery—the only one of its kind to date!

God provides peaceful sleep. The following quotes speak to this:

> In peace I will both lie down and sleep, for you alone, Lord, make me dwell in safety. (Ps. 4:8)

> It is in vain for you to rise up early, To sit up late, To eat the bread of sorrows; For so He gives his beloved sleep. (Ps. 127:2 NKJV)

> My son ... Keep sound wisdom and discretion ...
> Then you will walk safely in your way,
> And your foot will not stumble.
> When you lie down, you will not be afraid;
> Yes, you will lie down, and your sleep will be sweet. (Prov. 3:21–24 NKJV)

> Be anxious for nothing, but in everything, by prayer and supplication (petition), with thanksgiving, let your requests be made known to God; and the peace of God, which surpasses all understanding, will guard your hearts and your minds through Christ Jesus. (Phil. 4:6–7 NKJV)

Understanding and appreciating sleep as God's medicine is part of our faithfulness and trust in Him. This point is well illustrated in the below excerpt from French poet Charles Peguy's *The Portal of the Mystery of Hope* on the topic of sleep:

> I don't like the man who doesn't sleep,
> says God.
> Sleep is the friend of man,

3

Sleep is the friend of God.
Sleep is perhaps my most beautiful creation.
And I myself rested on the seventh day. ...
But they tell me that there are men
Who work well and sleep badly.
Who don't sleep. What a lack of
confidence in me.
It's almost worse than if they worked poorly but slept well.
I'm not talking, says God, about those men
Who don't work and don't sleep ...
I'm talking about those who work and who don't sleep.
I pity them. I hold it against them. A bit. They don't trust me.
As a child lays innocently in his mother's arms, thus they do
not lay.
Innocently in the arms of my Providence.
They have the courage to work. They don't have the courage
to do nothing.
They possess the virtue of work. They don't possess the virtue
of doing nothing.
Of relaxing. Of resting. Of sleeping.
Unhappy people, they don't know what's good.

The reader may argue this: What about the person who does
not sleep because he or she suffers from a sleep disorder?
And is this not pretty harsh and unloving of a God who is
love? Well, I believe Peguy is not referring to individuals with
sleep problems but is trying to describe God's chastising of
those workers who do not trust that God Himself is faithful to
provide, so as a result they habitually do not relax and sleep
at night.

Scripture says, "The sleep of a laboring man is sweet ..." (Eccl.
5:12). Sleep is one of the best medicines ever provided. Two other
medicines are food and water. Sleep is God's panacea for our

physical bodies. It is the choicest prescription ever written, yet is found in no pharmacy. There is no treatment that compares to sleep! God did not reserve His therapeutic gift of sleep for the special few (i.e., the wealthy or otherwise so privileged as to be the only ones able to afford it). In His infinite love, grace, and mercy, He bestowed it upon us all.

Two biblical references to sleep need further clarification. The first one is in Proverbs 20:13: "Do not love sleep, lest you come to poverty ..." This verse does not suggest that God or the writer of Proverbs was against sleep itself. The instruction is "not to love," be so enamored of, or idolize sleep that you become lazy. This is the same warning given about money in 1 Timothy 6:10: "For the love of money is a root of all kinds of evil, for which some have strayed from the faith in their greediness, and pierced themselves through with many sorrows." This verse is not against money itself; it says don't long for or worship money (or cultivate the desire to have more and more money) and the material excess that it can bring because this love of money can corrupt you and make you sin against Him.

The Big Sleep

The second biblical reference to sleep that must be clarified as being distinct from our daily slumber is related to the fact that humans have eternal spirits. It is only our current physical bodies that dies. Therefore, when sleep is referred to as death in the Bible, the description is only applicable to the body itself. When we die only our bodies are asleep. The following quotes support this idea:

> And the LORD said to Moses: "Behold, you will rest with your fathers ..." (Deut. 31:16 NKJV)

These things He said, and after that He said to them, "Our friend Lazarus sleeps, but I go that I may wake him up." Then His disciples said, "Lord, if he sleeps he will get well." However, Jesus spoke of his death, but they thought that He was speaking about taking rest in sleep." (John 11:11–13 NKJV)

David rested with his fathers. (1 Kings 11:21 NKJV)

Then Jehoshaphat rested with his ancestors and was buried with them in the City of David. (2 Chron. 21:1)

Now when David had served God's purpose in his own generation, he fell asleep; he was buried with his fathers and his body decayed. (Acts 13:36)

According to the Bible, permanent physical death does not exist. When a person dies in his or her sleep, most often it is said that the person died of natural causes. Yet I believe that these natural causes are really God declaring it is time. In 1939 author Raymond Chandler knew of this simile, comparing death to sleep when he entitled his first Detective Philip Marlowe novel *The Big Sleep.*

Just as the soul of the sleeper still exists (though oblivious to its external surroundings), in death the souls of humans are not extinct; they are only unaware of their earthly environment. In Ecclesiastics 9:5–6, Solomon asserted that the dead do not have knowledge of, nor reward for, anything transpiring "under the sun," that is, on earth.

It is written, "And many of those who sleep in the dust of the earth shall awake" (Dan. 12:2). This passage refers to the part of man that sleeps (the physical body, which has died), which is planted in the dust. Humans have eternal spirits. It is only the physical body that dies. When we die, we are only asleep (Deut. 31:16). A common Greek word for the sleep of death is *koimaomai* (Matt. 27:52), which is related to another Greek word *koimeterion*, which in antiquity meant sleeping room or burial place. It is from this word that we derive our word *cemetery*, the abode of dead bodies. Scripture says, "And the graves were opened; and many bodies of the saints who had fallen asleep were raised" (Matt. 27:52 NKJV).

Paul argues that Christ "is the firstfruits of those who have fallen asleep" (1 Cor. 15:20). This is a clear affirmation that Christ's bodily resurrection is heaven's pledge that we shall be raised similarly—the firstfruits being the initial harvest (cf. Ex. 23:16) and the guarantee of that which is to follow. As the Lord awoke from the dead, so shall we. All mankind will be born anew to eternal life ... so here sleep is renewal or revival— the word "revival" merely means "to live again."

"Our friend Lazarus has fallen asleep, but I go to awake him out of sleep" (John 11:11 UBV).

When we as believers die (pass on), sleep will serve a completely different remedy from the troubles and cares of this earthly existence; when we pass on, we will only temporarily fall asleep in Christ as we await His return. "'Blessed are the dead who die in the Lord from now on.' 'Yes,' says the Spirit, 'that they may rest from their labors, and their works follow them" (Rev. 14:13).

Then we will awake even more refreshed than during earthly life to share in God's heavenly banquet, before we are sent on to do the work ahead of us, which is to bring the day of God's glory closer to our world, and through it to the entire universe.

"Oh, death where is thy sting, oh grave where is thy victory?!" (1 Cor. 15:55 KJV).

A final word of encouragement as the sun sets on each day and rises to signal the start of a new day: let's not forget God, our Father and Creator. who by His Lordship alone has separated the Light from the darkness.

"This is the day that the Lord has made; We will rejoice and be glad in it" (Ps. 118:24 NKJV).

Please note, however, in the original languages of the Bible, the word "sleep" when referring to death was reserved only for believers who hoped to awake at the second coming of Christ.

Why Has God Made Sleep Necessary?

Sleep is not just a daily rest and relaxation time-out routine. It is an active state that is vitally important for our overall health and well-being. Jesus was speaking of the "sleep of death" when he told his disciples in John 11:11 that Lazarus, who had been very ill, had now fallen asleep. Yet they responded in the next verse, John 11:12, "Lord, if he sleeps, he will get better." The disciples knew of the great health benefits of sleep.

As far as we know, God designed the human body like no other in the universe. There is no machine or computer that could ever replace it in its entirety. Nor will God ever relinquish His sovereign authority to create a human body. Any attempt to do so will result in either failure or utter disaster. Yet we can look at the functions and activities that the body performs when we sleep as very similar to what a computer does in sleep mode or hibernate. In sleep mode the body and brain, like the desktop computer, are still turned on or active. The monitor is turned off, or the body is resting to conserve energy and to reduce wear and tear on certain components. The monitor powers down to use minimal current, while stopping the disk drives completely, though only after copying the current state of the computer to system RAM. Likewise, during sleep our memory tracks are consolidated and stored.

Sleep is intrinsically linked to health and illness. Sleep allows important physiologic changes to occur that are essential to maintaining one's mental, physical, and spiritual health and well-being. In addition sleep-related brain activities are daily brain servicing and reconditioning. God created this sleep medicine for us as a necessity in order to function and survive. Our bodies need sleep to heal. God wants us to have a good night's sleep in order that we may rise refreshed, relaxed, rejuvenated, and energetic—enthusiastic to start a new day. Inherent in this is His message to us that we are not self-sufficient. God alone is all-sufficient. He never sleeps nor slumbers, nor does he grow fatigued. This has always been and will always be. God is immutable.

"The everlasting God, the LORD, the Creator of the ends of the earth, neither faints nor is weary" (Isa. 40:28).

"He will not allow your foot slip; he who watches over you will not slumber. Indeed, he who keeps Israel will neither slumber nor sleep" (Ps. 121:3–4).

"For I am the LORD, I do not change" (Mal. 3:6 NKJV).

God created us for fellowship with Him and with others. When we allow ourselves to become sleep-deprived, we don't function as effectively and efficiently as we should. As a result we shortchange ourselves on sleep even more, trying to make up for lost time and poor efficiency. Some of the consequences observed in our spiritual and social life result in impaired mood and relationships, anxiety, depression, and increased alcohol use.

CHAPTER 2

———◉———

Medicine in the Bible

Webster's Universal College Dictionary defines "medicine" as: any substance used in the treatment of disease or illness. The definition is summarized as: a chemical substance, or any nonfood substance, used in the treatment, cure, prevention, or diagnosis of disease or to otherwise enhance physical or mental well-being or a nonfood substance intended to affect any function of the body. In the Greek language, *pharmakon*, from which we derive the English word "pharmaceutical," means a poison or medicine.

In the Old Testament (O.T.), one finds commands concerning the prevention and suppression of epidemics, suppression of sexually transmitted diseases and prostitution, sexual life, proper skin hygiene, baths, food, housing and clothing, labor rules and regulations, and appropriate discipline of the people. Many of these commands involve specifics on the Sabbath rest, circumcision, laws concerning food (interdiction of blood and pork), measures concerning menstruating and lying-in women and those suffering from gonorrhea, isolation of lepers, and hygiene of the camp.

Plants were the main source of healing remedies for healing in biblical times. Balm, figs, hyssop, and oil are the only plant products mentioned in the Bible with reference to healing. In Jeremiah 8:22 the prophet cries, "Is there no balm in Gilead, Is there no physician there?" Isaiah, in chapter 38 verse 21, prescribes "a lump of figs" prepared and applied as a poultice for King Hezekiah's boil. In Isaiah 1:6 he speaks of "bruises and sores and bleeding wounds" that "have not been closed, or bound up, or soothed with ointment." Of particular interest is the herb hyssop, which the ancient Hebrew called *azob*, meaning "holy herb." They used it as a cleansing herb for temples and other sacred places. It was also used for purification rites. But the ancient Romans used hyssop for protection from the plague and to repel insects. In ancient Greece the physicians Galen and Hippocrates used hyssop to treat inflammations of the throat and chest, pleurisy, and other bronchial complaints. Although hyssop has some antimicrobial and antiviral properties (1 Kings 4:33; Ps. 51:7; John 19:29), the German Commission E has not approved this herb for any medicinal purposes. References to the hyssop plant in the Gospels of Matthew and Mark use the general term *kalamos*, which is translated "reed" or "stick."

Medicinal forms of treatment were rarely mentioned in the New Testament; rather, accounts of miraculous healing or curing were the norm. Most cures were from natural diseases. The four gospels contain approximately thirty-five instances of Jesus' miraculous healing of individuals and groups of people. The first New Testament account of Jesus' healing is recorded in Matthew 4:23: "And Jesus went about all Galilee, teaching in their synagogues, preaching the gospel of the kingdom, and healing all kinds of sickness and all kinds of disease among the people." Jesus' miraculous healing included cleansing lepers, healing a man with dropsy (edema most often related to congestive heart failure), another with a withered hand, and a woman with a hemorrhage. He also healed the blind, deaf, lame, and epileptic and cast out demons. This miraculous cleansing or healing power was also bestowed on the twelve apostles—"power against unclean spirits, to cast them out, to heal all manner of sickness and all manner of disease." The blind received their sight, the lame walked, lepers were cleansed and healed, and the deaf received their hearing.

CHAPTER 3

Theories of Sleep

From the beginning of recorded history, humans have been fascinated and intrigued by the phenomenon of sleep, culminating in the emergence of many theories and speculations on: "What is sleep?" and "Why do we need this daily activity?"

Sleep Theories from Classical Antiquity

Many prominent Greek philosophers, authors and physicians being quite cerebral (intellectual) thinkers believed sleep to be a pathological condition suppressing the part of the soul that houses rational thought and behavior including suppresion of higher cognitive functions such as the ability to reason, yet lower physical functions remained active to digest food and produce "vapors". However, their Latin counterparts often believed the mind was still awake and active during sleep. The early Christian author-philosophers, Augustine and Tertullian interpreted sleep as evidence of the eternal existence of the soul (Dossey 2013).

Cerebral Hypoperfusion Theory

This reduced cerebral flow view of sleep onset was derived from Alcmaeon of Croton, a Greek medical writer and physiologist of the sixth century BC, who proposed that sleep is the result of blood draining away from the head (or in some interpretations: away from the surface of the body) and then being diverted to other larger parts ("blood-flowing" vessels) of the body, especially the gut. When the cerebral blood level depletes to a certain amount, a person loses consciousness, or what Alcmaeon called 'sleep'. A person awakes from sleep when the blood diffuses back throughout the body. Cerebral hypoperfusion during sleep in certain sleep disorders or medical conditions has been shown to affect the quality of one's sleep. However, to date, there is no evidence that this is a contributing factor in normal sleep onset or duration.

Cardiocerebral Vapors Circulation Theory

Aristotle, the reknown fourth century BC Greek philosopher, argued in his works "De Somno et Vigilia" (On Sleeping and Waking) and "Topics" 145b14-16 that after we eat, our food is carried to the center of the stomach and digested by the heat of the heart. This digestive process causes hot "vapors" (or "exhalations") to ascend to and collect in the brain from the stomach to a higher temperature in the head, and the head becomes heavy. Then as the brain cools and the mind shuts down, these vapors condense and descend back down into the heart sensory organ and related lesser sensory organs, cooling them, thereby producing the induction of sleep. He asserted that spells of sleep (non-pathological epilepsy) follow eating because a large quantity of dense liquids and solid matter weighs a person down and causes one to nod; and by the return of cooled vapors to the heart, the hot vapors in the heart are repulsed, causing the sensory faculties to fail, and thus sleep ensues (Dossey 2013).

Alemaeon and Aristotle's theories are not supported by known human anatomy or cerebrovascular and cardiovascular circulation. In addition, Aristotle's theory doesn't explain how and why individuals who are completely fasting or who are simply on a liquid fast can still sleep normally.

Toxin or Waste-Induced Sleep Theory

This pathological toxins view asserts that sleep is the result of daytime waste by-products, which gradually accumulate to induce a temporary stupor or sleep.

Several facts clearly refute this assertion:

- Sleep can occur during any part of the day or night.
- We know that waste products are produced by the body on a continual basis. There is no evidence that our excretory organs—the kidney (urine), colon (feces), liver (metabolic breakdown of products and toxins), lungs (carbon dioxide from respiration), and skin (sweat)—produce the greater amount of their waste products or reach some critical mass by day's end, thereby inducing sleep. Sweat is the only waste product that is secreted at night. Except for problems with urination or defecation, all other waste products are removed only during wakefulness (the vast majority of carbon dioxide is removed during respiration when you are awake engaging in normal intermittent deep breathing). Furthermore, we know that for healthy individuals sleep is innate and they are easily awakened—which indicates that we are not intoxicated by body toxins or poisons as we sleep.
- Conjoined twins although rare share some of the same circulatory (blood and lymph) system and may share some of the same organs and neuro circuitry - all depending upon where they are connected, yet if they survive, it has been noted that one twin is able to sleep while the other twin can be fully awake and active.

Early Industrial Age Sleep Theory: Fetal Regression, 1856–1939

The famous Austrian psychiatrist Sigmund Freud, traditionally referred to as the father of psychoanalysis, contended that sleep is a psychological phenomenon involving a subconscious desire or motivation to retreat from life's difficulties and stressors. He suggested that man developed the sleep mechanism to accommodate this subconscious longing to retreat to the security of fetal life. He also postulated that we dream during sleep because we are acting out wish fulfillments of internally repressed ideas and feelings that cannot be expressed during wakefulness, thereby dreams protecting us from sleep disruption.

All of the above theories (some for various obvious reasons) have not been supported by the scientific method, except for Aristotle, who was on to something when he related cooling body temperature to sleep induction. In fact, we still have the same sleep cycle that is evidenced in all the historical records of antiquity. Since sleep is God's medicine, we will probably never (in this life) fully understand it. As Gary Webster writes in his 1957 book *The Wonders of Man*, "(sleep is) a nightly miracle that baffles science." Healthy sleep is evidence that "every good and perfect gift" comes from God above.

Modern Schools of Thought

There are three modern schools of thought on why we sleep:

Restorative or Repair—Sleep serves a biological and physiologic need. Sleep enables the body and brain to rejuvenate, rest and restore energy levels, and repair, replenishing key areas of the brain or body that are depleted during the day. Specifically, during sleep the brain performs vital housekeeping tasks, such as organizing long-term memory, integrating new information and allowing the mind to sort out past, present, and future activities and feelings. In addition, there is repairing and renewing of tissue and, nerve cells and replenishing of needed biochemical substances.

Adaptive—Sleep evolved as a protective adaptation for humans. It was necessary for our survival. It prevented our ancestors from wasting their physical and mental energy and exposing themselves to the dangers of predators and other pitfalls while roaming around after dark fall. For both nomadic and hunter-gatherer societies, finding food in the daytime and hiding or staying undercover at night was easier and more protective. Humans sleep at times that maximize their safety, given their physical capacities and limitations and their chosen habitats. In addition, the amount and quality of sleep achieved is directly proportional to the amount and quality of each day's productivity.

Homeostasis—The sleep drive has a homeostatic mechanism that defines the relationship between wakefulness and sleep. It is a function of the duration of wakefulness. It helps prevent the healthy individual from becoming dangerously sleep-deprived and after a long day of mental and physical work prepares you for sleep.

As we can see from the above sampling, over the past 2,500 years, starting with the days of Aristotle, there have been many theories regarding the origin and nature of sleep, but to date there is no universally accepted theory on any aspect of sleep.

CHAPTER 4

---◈---

Anthropology of Sleep

Western treatments for sleep mainly focus on medications, establishing a presleep routine and other measures, some of which can be highly effective. Yet cross-culturally, there is a significant variation in sleep patterns and habits. The two main differences across different societies revolve around the availability of artificial light sources and communal sleep. Ekirch in his 2006 book *"At Day's Close..."* stated (as also did other sleep historians) that the primary difference is that pre-artificial light societies had more fragmented sleep patterns. Thus, the boundaries between sleeping and waking tended to be blurred in these societies. People might go to sleep far more quickly after the sun goes down, but they would then wake up several times throughout the night, punctuating their sleep with periods of wakefulness, perhaps lasting several hours.

Artificial light has been plentiful in the industrialized Western world since at least the mid-nineteenth century, and sleep patterns have changed significantly everywhere that this lighting has been introduced. In many well-lit societies, this lighting, along with advances in modern transportation and electronic communication, have allowed activities of daily living to proceed nearly around the clock, despite the cloak of darkness. Parts of the night have thus been transformed into daytime.

Some societies show pronounced differences in sleeping patterns. Some may display a fragmented sleep pattern, in which people sleep at various times during the day and night for shorter periods. Others have changed from one pattern to the next over the course of time. In many nomadic or hunter-gatherer societies still in existence today, people sleep off and on throughout the day or night depending on what is happening. Many Mediterranean and South American cultures have a *siesta*, a period during the afternoon in which people sleep.

Historically most humans slept clustered together with friends, animals, parents, and children. Multiple-room dwellings for the masses first occurred less than two hundred years ago. Yet around the world today, most people still live in one-room dwellings, where most activities of daily living take place. In almost every culture today, sleeping partners are strongly regulated by societal standards. In most societies infants sleep with an adult, while older children sleep with younger siblings. This communal sleep, also known as co-sleep, was and still is considered safer for various reasons: help is readily available in case of an emergency; and it is part of the nurturing process for children. These societies found that group sleeping reduced the risk of spirit loss, which is especially common when a person dreams.

In almost all societies, sleeping partners are strongly regulated by customary social standards. Depending on sleep groupings, sleep may be an actively social time, with little or no constraints on noise or activity. In some societies people sleep with at least one other person, often many, or with animals. For example, people might only sleep with their spouses, immediate or extended family, their children, children of a certain age or specific gender, peers of a certain gender, peers of equal social rank, or with no one at all. In other societies people rarely sleep with anyone except one with whom they have a most intimate relationship, such as a spouse. In Mayan (Guatemalan) and Japanese cultures, mothers do not believe in separate sleeping quarters for infants, small children, and parents. In the United States, Hispanics, African-Americans, and Appalachians (the latter population reputedly has had a long-term resistance to social change) cosleep with their infants more often than their European-American counterparts, who cosleep primarily when their infants are perceived to have sleeping problems.

In the past ten years there has been considerable research on co-sleeping or bed-sharing. At one month infants are still very neurologically immature and overall development is slower than in later months. One outcome of this neurological immaturity and slower development is that very small young infants are not able to consolidate periods of sleep. Survey research published by McKenna and Volpe in 2007 found that infant sleep development is significantly effected in the first few years of life by a diversity of sleeping arrangements and practices. Their research outlined the importance of maternal proximity and breast-feeding in regulating infant sleep physiology. McKenna purports that mother-infant physical contact probably assists in regulating the baby's body temperature, breathing patterns, arousal patterns, cortisol levels, and sleep architecture (sleep patterns). These authors also emphasized that family values and social relationships should be respected in order to achieve an effective public health approach to creating safe sleep environments for infants and children.

Since McKenna's study the United States Health and Human Services Agency has developed the Safe to Sleep® program. The principles and guidelines of this program do not support or advocate co-sleeping for infants younger than one year old. In fact, this program emphasizes that safe sleep is only in the supine position (on the baby's back) from birth until the time when an infant is able to safely and completely roll over from left to right or right to left independently from a supine to a prone position (on the baby's stomach and abdomen) and back to supine. Until that time an infant should never be allowed to sleep in the prone position or on his/her side. Additional safe sleep tips and habits for small infants are provided in Chapter 11 – Sleep Throughout the Life Cycle.

CHAPTER 5

---◆---

Sleep Architecture (Sleep Patterns) and Physiology

God designed our bodies to partake of the necessary-for-survival, essential-to-life medicine called sleep. Our bodies are designed for sleep to come effortlessly. God created our internal biological clocks and circadian rhythms to respond to the way He created the earth on which we live. He draws the curtains of darkness; and then He comes and says, "Sleep, sleep, my child; I give thee sleep." He hides the sun until daybreak.

Researchers have concluded that sleep is an active, complex, and dynamic state that greatly influences our waking hours. They also realize that we must understand sleep to better understand the brain. Yet this chapter, out of necessity and the overall purpose of this book, will scarcely scratch the surface of the highly complex initiating and control mechanisms involved in sleep. The sleep architecture described below is that of a normal healthy adult person.

Humans are diurnal beings designed to be active during the daytime and to sleep at night. Sleep structure has distinct stages and rhythms. Sleep is defined as a cycle with five stages. The cycle of sleep and wakefulness is regulated by the brain stem, thalamus, external stimuli, and various hormones produced by the hypothalamus. Sleep is controlled by our internal biological clock, which in turn controls our circadian rhythm and homeostatic sleep drive.

At night the neurotransmitter serotonin usually starts off the sleep cycle, leading to the production of the hormone called melatonin. Melatonin secreted by the pineal gland peaks at night and induces sleep; the informational signal for the pineal gland to secrete melatonin comes from the body's internal biological clock. This clock is named the suprachiasmatic nucleus or SCN. It is a pair of pinhead-size brain structures (in the hypothalamus) that together contain about 20,000 neurons. The approximate twenty-four-hour cyclical secretion of melatonin from the pineal gland establishes the circadian rhythm. Our circadian sleep rhythms are regular changes in sleep characteristics that occur in the course of a day or approximately twenty-four-hour period ("circadian" is Latin for "around a day").

In the morning, light that reaches photoreceptors in the retina creates signals that travel along the optic nerve to the SCN. In the presence of light, the SCN then sends messages to the pineal gland that instruct it to cease secreting melatonin, which promotes wakefulness and increased alertness by signaling body temperature to rise.

Disruptions of the circadian rhythms often lead to common sleep-related problems, such as jet lag and shift work-related daytime somnolence. The SCN is very sensitive to the presence or absence of light. This may explain why daytime sleep without the intervention of conditions that simulate nighttime is often less restful than nighttime sleep.

There are two periods within our circadian rhythm when we express our strongest drive for sleep: the first and the strongest between 2:00 a.m. and 4:00 a.m. and then a second between 1:00 p.m. and 3:00 p.m.

Most individuals' biological body clocks work on an approximate twenty-five-hour lunar cycle rather than a twenty-four-hour solar one. Our internal circadian clocks normally follow the twenty-four-hour cycle of the sun, rather than our body clocks, because sunlight or bright light can reset the SCN. Specifically, in most humans the natural day length of the circadian clock is approximately twenty-four hours and ten minutes; therefore, the clock must be entrained (reset) to match the day length of the external environmental clock (that is, the day/night cycle). Light is the cue that synchronizes the internal biological clock to the environmental cycle. Since most people are exposed to regular cycles of day and night, the pineal gland automatically adapts to the length of a twenty-four-hour solar cycle. Our biological clocks are reset daily, but they can only shift about two or three hours per day and only at certain times of the day.

Most totally blind individuals, especially those blind from birth, experience lifelong sleeping problems because their retinas are unable to detect light. These individuals display periodic insomnia and a circadian-rhythm sleep disorder very similar to permanent jet lag because their circadian rhythms follow their internal biological clock, rather than a twenty-four-hour one governed by sunlight. Unfortunately, because their retinas are unable to detect light, studies to date have not shown that an intervention such as bright-light therapy is of much benefit for these individuals. Manufactured in various forms bright-light therapy is a modality that provides a level of light which matches that of outdoors light shortly after sunrise or before sunset. In addition, even for the sighted, individual response to light therapy varies widely.

Sleep also triggers the release of hormones. During the deep sleep of the first few hours of sleep, human growth hormone (HGH) is actively produced, helping to regenerate the body. The pituitary gland produces HGH for muscle repair, mucus membrane healing, and tissue growth and repair. It also helps the body to sustain energy levels, promotes lean muscle mass, and helps prevent unnecessary fat gain as we age. Deep sleep can be viewed as "beauty sleep" because during this stage protein synthesis is increased yet breakdown is decreased; cellular growth is enhanced, and damages from UV light and stress are repaired. Sleep promotes the release of progesterone, which promotes fertility.

Concomitant other physical changes in body temperature, hormone secretion, urine production, and blood pressure occur because light-induced signals from the SCN travel to the brain regions governing these activities. Prolactin, testosterone, and human growth hormone demonstrate circadian rhythms, with maximal secretion during the night. Normal pubertal changes occur in the body as we mature because a decrease in melatonin levels signals the body to begin puberty and the maturation process. But if peak levels of melatonin stay high, puberty will not begin. Therefore, prepubescent children who take melatonin for sleep may be at risk for delaying their sexual maturation.

The second event that influences sleep is related to the buildup of adenosine. Brain cells give off adenosine as a waste product that builds up during the day in the basal forebrain. Inside the forebrain adenosine acts to inhibit brain cells that normally promote wakefulness and play key roles in brain function. When one eventually falls asleep at night, brain function relaxes, brain cells work less hard, and adenosine is taken back into brain cells, relieving its pressure on the wakefulness neurocircuit of the brain. Some researchers believe that this adenosine buildup is the neurochemical basis for our homeostatic sleep drive. The homeostatic sleep drive is a function of how much wakefulness a person has experienced. The longer one stays awake, the stronger and more intense this drive makes our need for sleep. This drive is reduced in intensity by sleeping.

The stages of sleep were originally defined by studying the process of sleep using primarily three measurements. *Gross brain wave or electrical activity* was measured using the electroencephalogram or EEG. The *body's muscle tone* was measured using the electromyogram or EMG. The third measurement, *gross eye movement,* was recorded using the electrooculogram or EOG. Together these three measurements came to be known as polysomnography, the technological basis for all sleep lab analyses. Measurable characteristic differences in these three measurements define each stage of sleep. Modern sleep studies also include continuous pulse oximetry (monitoring of the patient's heart rate, respiratory rate, and blood oxygen level), monitoring limb, chin, and chest movements and electrocardiogram. Another parameter studied in sleep laboratories is sleep latency, as assessed by the Multiple Sleep Latency Test (MSLT). The MSLT is used to diagnose narcolepsy and idiopathic hypersomnia. Technicians in the sleep laboratory or clinic maintain logs that include documentation of patient body position and body activity.

Sleep is a progressive slowing of brain-wave activity until rapid eye movement (REM) sleep occurs. There are five phases of sleep. Stages 1, 2, 3, and 4 are called non-REM or NREM sleep, delta or slow-wave, or quiet sleep. Collectively, stages 1 through 4 of NREM comprise 75–80 percent of sleep. The fifth phase of sleep is called rapid eye movement (REM) sleep or "paradoxical sleep" (REM is called paradoxical sleep because in this stage of sleep, brain-wave activity is similar to an awakened state, but a person exhibits muscle atonia (loss of muscle tone) and a person's eyes actually move quickly under the eyelids while the brain is exercising. During REM sleep, muscles that move the eyes, and those involved in breathing, continue to function, but most of the body's other voluntary muscles are stopped. This naturally reversible Deep R or REM sleep paralysis (lack of muscle movement except for eye movements, respiration, and the movement of the tiny bones in the middle ear) protects individuals from injuring themselved by unconsciously acting out their dreams while in REM sleep. For those not suffering from a sleep disorder, muscle control, and movement resume before becoming consciously awake.

The stages of sleep progress in a cycle from stage 1 to the end of the cycle with REM sleep, and then the cycle starts over again at stage 1. A sleep cycle is defined as one complete progression through these stages of sleep. A sleep cycle on the average takes ninety to 110 minutes to complete. Normally, there are approximately five sleep cycles per night.

Stage 1 (light theta-wave sleep) of NREM sleep occurs while a person is falling asleep. During stage 1 of sleep, sleep induction begins: the body temperature drops, muscles relax, and the eyes often deviate from side to side. Drowsiness ensues, and we slip into a loss of awareness of our surroundings and sleep begins. There is no medication on the market anywhere in the world that, when given alone, can induce so tranquil a transition into sleep. What a wonderful prelude! This stage represents about 3 to 5 percent of a normal healthy adult sleep time. Most people awakened after sleeping more than a few minutes usually cannot recall the last few minutes before they fell asleep. This sleep-related form of amnesia is the reason why telephone calls or conversations are often forgotten that took place in the middle of the night. In addition, this form of amnesia explains why we often do not remember our alarms going off in the morning if we go right back to sleep after turning them off. If awakened in sleep stage 1 or 2, individuals will often remark that they had not been asleep at all.

Stage 2 (true light theta-wave sleep), called "non-REM" (non-rapid eye movement) NREM sleep is the start of "true" sleep. This stage represents about 45 to 50 percent (the majority) of total adult sleep time. As one drifts into this stage of NREM sleep, the higher brain centers begin to rest and quiet, enabling a person to enter the third stage of NREM, deep sleep or quiet sleep. Gamma-amino butyric acid (GABA) is a naturally occurring neurochemical substance in the brain manufactured from amino acids that is associated with sleep patterns, specifically sleep initiation. GABA has a calming effect. During this stage a person's EEG will show distinctive waveforms that are the hallmark of NREM sleep, called *sleep spindles* (brief bursts of fast oscillatory brain activity) generated by GABA-nergic neurons and *K complexes* (composed of large positive and negative waves that stand out from the background on the EEG tracing and often occur in response to environmental or external stimuli, such as sounds and touch). Researchers at the University of California Berkley (Mander, Santhanam, Saletin, & Walker, 2011) demonstrated that sleep spindles are reliable predictors of refreshment of one's ability to learn.

Stage 3 (early deep delta or slow-wave sleep) and stage 4 (deep slow-wave sleep) of NREM sleep are the deepest levels of human sleep and represent 15 to 20 percent of adult sleep time. There is no significant division between these two stages except, typically, stage 3 has less than 50 percent of the waves as delta waves and stage 4 has more than 50 percent of the waves as delta waves and is thus a more intense deep sleep. The mind and body are quietest during these stages of sleep. The body is still, breathing is shallow and regular, the body's muscles are loose, and one is "out like a light." As sleep ensues, activity in nearly all parts of the brain slow, but the area that slows the greatest is the prefrontal cortex (the area of the brain that is responsible for logical thinking, reasoning, problem-solving, and planning). It is very difficult to wake someone up from these stages, which together are called deep sleep. Renewal and restoration of the body is accomplished during stages 3 and 4 of sleep. In the normal adult, deep sleep (stages 3 and 4) lasts an approximate total of four to five hours.

During the first sleep cycle after about ninety minutes in quiet sleep (stages 1–4), the brain begins to become more active, norepinephrine and serotonin levels (which help us focus attention and solve problems when we are awake) taper off, and acetylcholine turns on. Acetylcholine is associated with memory formation in the awake and sleep states. This shift in hormone levels brings a person out of deep sleep (stages 3 and 4) and into light sleep (stages 1 and 2) next to allow REM sleep or active sleep to occur.

Stage 5, rapid eye movement (REM) sleep, as just stated, usually begins about ninety minutes after one falls asleep (in certain individuals this time frame can be as short as seventy minutes). The first REM sleep period is part of an important measure called REM latency (the duration of sleep between when an individual first falls asleep and the onset of the first REM sleep period). REM latency when reduced is a significant clinical marker of several psychiatric disorders. REM sleep alternates with NREM sleep about every ninety minutes throughout the night. PGO spikes on the EEG (bursts of electric energy fired from neurons located in the pons (P) region of the brain stem, through the geniculate (G) body, and to the occipital cortex (O), are a distinct neurophysiologic feature of REM sleep. REM periods increase in length over the course of the night. REM accounts for 20 to 25 percent of total adult sleep time.

When REM sleep begins, all the areas of the brain that were turned off in NREM sleep Gear up except one: the logical, reasoning portion of the prefrontal cortex. In REM sleep the serotonin system turns itself off. Remember, serotonin helps thoughts flow in a fairly orderly, coherent manner so that we can focus and solve problems. During this stage of sleep, individuals dream and stir, turn over, and may even adjust their bedcovers without fully awakening. One may also awaken during this stage, go to the bathroom, return to bed, and fall back into a deep sleep.

The first cycle of sleep proceeds in progression from stage 1 through 4, to REM sleep. All subsequent cycles of sleep proceed as alternating cycles of light and deep sleep. These subsequent cycles progress from REM sleep through stages 2 and 3, ending with REM sleep. This cycle pattern continues every couple hours throughout the night, so that a typical adult may spend an average of six hours in quiet sleep (stages 1–4) and two hours in active sleep (REM). It was determined through the analysis of the normal cyclical pattern of sleep that the average adult needs about eight hours of sleep a night. However, if our REM sleep is disrupted one night, our bodies don't follow this normal sleep cycle progression the next time we doze off. Instead, we often slip directly into REM sleep, going through extended periods of REM until we catch up on this stage of sleep.

Sleep cycles vary with a person's age, and sleep patterns vary greatly by age. In early adolescence, teens experience a natural shift in their circadian rhythms that are in conflict with the early awake times that school schedules mandate. Children and adolescents have longer periods of Stage 3 and

Stage 4 NREM sleep than do middle-age or older adults. Teens characteristically experience delayed sleep onset, wherein they typically do not feel sleepy until around 11:00 p.m. and prefer to sleep longer in the mornings until about 9:00 a.m. Total REM sleep declines with age. Infants spend about 50 percent of their sleep time in REM and the other 50 percent in NREM sleep. Adults spend about 20 percent of their sleep time in REM and 80 percent in NREM sleep. The elderly spend less than 15 percent of their sleep time in REM sleep. In addition, older adults tend to develop advanced sleep onset, which means that on the average they go to bed and arise earlier than their middle-aged counterparts. Furthermore, older adults tend to awaken more often from sleep. In light of these differences, when evaluating a patient for a sleep disorder primary care providers should take into account the patient's age.

CHAPTER 6

Sleep Loss, Sleep Deprivation, and Sleep Debt

Sleep experts maintain that most adults need between seven and nine hours of sleep each night for optimum functioning, health, and safety. When we don't get sufficient enough sleep on a daily basis, we will accumulate a sleep debt that can be difficult to pay back if it becomes too great. The stress of improper sleep may not show up right away, but its accumulative negative effects are apparent nonetheless. One will eventually see the effects in terms of premature aging, degenerative processes within the body, and early death.

Excessive daytime sleepiness is a major US public health concern often associated with significant interference with daily activities, including cognitive functioning, on-the-job performance, and productivity. In fact, poor-quality sleep can lead to daytime fatigue. The safety record of all forms of transportation has been negatively affected by the societal pervasiveness of excessive daytime sleepiness. This excessive daytime sleepiness can spill over to difficulty with night time driving due to accumulated sleep debt. Surveys of transportation records consistently reveal that fatal traffic accidents peak on the day after the change in daylight savings time.

Consequences of Long-Term Sleep Loss

A broad array of health problems are associated with prolonged sleep loss, medically known as "chronic cumulative sleep loss." Slow-wave sleep (deep sleep) is essential for health. Individuals with chronic insomnia are at risk for early death. Chronic deep-sleep deprivation can even lead to death. Here's a potential question for future research: Is this the reason why slow-wave deep sleep is nearly absent in most people over age sixty-five as these individuals age and prepare for dying? Specifically, sleep deprivation has been linked to health problems, such as obesity and high blood pressure, negative mood and behavior, decreased productivity, and safety issues in the home, at work, and on the highways.

During sleep, levels of cytokines decline, but after one day of sleep deprivation, levels of IL-6 cytokines are increased. High levels of these cytokines indicate that inflammatory processes have been geared up somewhere in the body. Elevated levels have been linked to cardiovascular disease and metabolic syndrome. Metabolic syndrome is a common disorder consisting of a cluster of abnormalities that include insulin resistance, dyslipidemia, and hypercoagulability. Studies have reported that patient sleep deprivation due to elevated noise levels can increase cortisol levels and an individual's heart and respiratory rates. Elevated cholesterol levels are also associated with increased risk for cancer, Alzheimer's disease, type 2 diabetes, and atherosclerosis. Chronically sleep-deprived individuals are more likely to have impaired glucose tolerance tests and demonstrate decreased sensitivity to insulin (Morselli, Leproult, Balbo, and Spiegel 2010; Byberg, Hansen, Christensen, Vistisen, Aadahl, Linneberg, & Witte 2012).

Most individuals develop cognitive deficits from chronic sleep deprivation after only a few nights of reduced sleep quality or quantity. Forgetfulness and difficulty concentrating are common. In addition, there are important health-related consequences from sleep loss, including increased susceptibility to common viral illnesses and depression, along with increased risk of obesity, diabetes, heart disease, gastrointestinal disorders, and menstrual irregularities. Sleep deprivation can cause increased sensitivity to pain, stomach upset, and decreased tolerance to annoying or bothersome stimuli.

Chronic lack of sleep can substantially impair the immune system. A depressed or impaired immune system can increase one's cancer risk. Insufficient sleep affects growth hormone secretion, which is linked to obesity; as the amount of hormone secretion decreases, the chance for weight gain increases. Research has also shown that insufficient sleep over time weakens the immune system and impairs the body's ability to use insulin, and thereby increases the risk for chronic health conditions such as diabetes and obesity (Broussard, Ehrmann, Van Cauter, Tasali and Brady 2012; Engeda, Mezuk, Ratliff, and Ning 2013). Scientific studies are continuing to reveal significant correlations between poor or insufficient sleep and disease.

Sleep is postulated to help the body conserve energy and other bodily resources that the immune system needs to mount a defense. The production of the hormone melatonin (which mostly occurs at night) enhances immune responses, increases resistance to viral infections, and inhibits tumor growth. How the immune system functions at night defines a specific role of sleep in the formation of immunological memory. While one is sleeping, the body's immune system increases its natural killer T-cell production to fight off infection. Neurons that control sleep interact closely with the immune system. This probably occurs because cytokines, the immuno-molecular proteins that our immune system produces to fight infections, are powerful sleep-inducing chemicals. During an infection these blood cytokines, also known as interleukins, are naturally occurring glycoproteins that mediate and regulate immune responses, increase to activate the immune system, and defend against infection (specifically interleukin-6, called IL-6). Infectious diseases tend to make us feel sleepy because these inflammatory cytokines also cause symptoms of sleepiness (Besedovsky, Lange, and Born 2012).

Blood pressure usually falls during the sleep cycle; however, interrupted sleep can adversely affect this normal decline, leading to hypertension and cardiovascular problems. The ongoing Nurses' Health Study (currently in its third incarnation) showed a 45 percent increase in the risk of fatal and nonfatal myocardial infarction (heart attack) among those who slept five or less hours a night. In 2006 Columbia University researchers reviewed the 1982 health surveys of middle-aged people residing in the United States and follow-up surveys published ten years later, in 1992. Review of these surveys revealed that over 4,800 individuals reported sleeping five or fewer hours per night each week. If their reports were accurate, these individuals were possibly increasing their risk of high blood pressure. Why? The prevailing thought is that they may have been depriving their bodies of a much-needed rest from cardiovascular system activity.

According to an analysis of the 2002 National Health Interview Survey published in 2006, for the 31,044 adults participating in the survey, insomnia and trouble sleeping were most often associated with high blood pressure, heart failure, anxiety, and depression. Prior to this survey, the prevailing thought was that insomnia was quite prevalent on its own, but only 4 percent of the people who said they had insomnia stated that they had it without any of these conditions.

According to the Mayo Clinic™, one's risk of insomnia is greater if:

- you are a woman. Women are much more likely to experience insomnia. Hormonal shifts during the menstrual cycle and in menopause may play a role. During menopause, night sweats and hot flashes often disturb sleep. Insomnia is also common with pregnancy.
- you are older than age sixty. Because of changes in sleep patterns and health, insomnia increases with age.
- you have a mental health disorder. Many disorders—including depression, anxiety, bipolar disorder, and post-traumatic stress disorder—disrupt sleep. Early-morning awakening is a classic symptom of depression.
- you are under a lot of stress. Stressful events can cause temporary insomnia. And major or long-lasting stress, such as the death of a loved one or a divorce, can lead to chronic insomnia. Being poor or unemployed also increases the risk.
- you work nights or changing shifts. Working at night or frequently changing shifts increases your risk of insomnia.
- you travel long distances. Jet lag from traveling across multiple time zones can cause insomnia. (Retrieved June 18, 2013, from http://www.mayoclinic.org/diseases-conditions/insomnia/basics/risk-factors/con-20024293)

Realizing that satisfactory sleep is a universal imperative for healthy human functioning and survival, the National

Sleep Foundation (NSF) sponsors annual telephone survey polls on the sleep and sleep habits of Americans. Each year a different demographic group is the focus of the survey. The first international poll, conducted in 2013, comparing the sleep in the United States with sleep in three other industrialized nations will not be covered in this book.

Surveys conducted by the NSF reveal that each year at least 40 million Americans suffer from chronic, long-term sleep disorders, and an additional 20 million experience occasional sleeping problems. Sleep problems are, in fact, the second most commonly reported medical complaint, the first being pain. To date more than seventy sleep disorders have been described. These disorders and the resultant sleep deprivation that they cause interfere with on-the-job performance, driving safety, and social activities. They also account for an estimated $16 billion in medical costs each year, while the indirect costs due to lost productivity and other factors are inarguably much greater. Other than the lack of food or water, no other deficiency in life besides sleep loss can cause more ubiquitous and wide-ranging negative effects in so short an amount of time.

A review of the NSF Sleep in America polls over the past decade reveal some startling revelations about Americans' sleep habits and day-to-day functioning in the setting of sleep loss. All the following information and additional detailed information on NSF polls can be found by visiting their website at www. nationalsleepfoundation.org/sleep-polls-data.

The National Sleep Foundation 2003 poll – Sleep and Aging questioned respondents about their mood, outlook on life, cognitive function, social involvement, exercise frequency, and financial security. In general, those who assessed themselves positively in these areas were more likely to sleep seven to nine hours each night, rate their sleep quality as excellent or very good, and report fewer sleep problems and sleep disorder diagnoses.

The National Sleep Foundation 2005 poll – Adult Sleep Habits and Styles revealed that on the average, 71 percent of American adults get only 6.9 hours of sleep a night, slightly less than what many sleep professionals recommend: a total of seven to nine hours each night. Seventy-five percent of adults reported at least one frequent sleep problem symptom, most commonly either waking up feeling unrefreshed or waking up often during the night. Despite these symptoms on the average 75 percent of respondents having at least one frequent sleep problem reported that they ignore their symptoms, and only 20 percent or less of these individuals believed that they actually had a sleep problem. Many adults often reported feeling tired, fatigued, or not feeling up to par the next day; yet, most did not take steps to improve their quality of sleep or to get a more optimum amount of sleep.

Four percent of respondents who drove or had a license to drive reported having had an accident or near-accident while driving because they were too tired or dozed off at the wheel. Driving while drowsy is equated to driving with a .05 percent blood alcohol (BA) level. Many may think, "So what? This level is still below the .08 percent DUI level set by most states," but there is a problem with stopping the analysis right here. Drivers with BA levels just below .08 percent, although not legally driving drunk, are to varying degrees under the influence and are still awake. They can sometimes use their reflexes, impaired though they may be, to prevent an accident, often leaving skid marks all over the road. Traffic accident investigators have deduced many times that the driver in a fatal or near-fatal accident probably fell asleep at the wheel because there were no skid marks on the road. To address this problem, the NSF has established a national Drowsy Driver education program. More information can be obtained by visiting www.drowsydriver.org.

According to the National Sleep Foundation 2006 poll –Teens and Sleep, in general, most adolescents need at least eight and a half hours of sleep each night with only a few minor interruptions in order to perform well in the daytime. Inadequate sleep and poor sleep habits are very common, especially among adolescents and young adults. Adolescents defined in this poll as being between eleven and seventeen years of age reported getting the optimum nine hours of sleep on school nights only 20 percent of the time. Forty-five percent of adolescents reported that they got less than eight hours of sleep on school nights. More than 50 percent of teens reported they knew they were not getting enough sleep in order to feel their best. Adolescents who on most school nights slept much less than the optimum in order to feel their best were more likely to be night owls and to have sleep-deprivation after effects such as feeling cranky or irritable with resultant difficulty getting along with their families, or they felt too tired to engage in exercise or other physical activities.

In addition, 51 percent of adolescents reported driving while feeling drowsy during the past year, which probably still contributed significantly to teen automobile accidents. The poll revealed that nine out of ten parents believed that their adolescent children were getting enough sleep at least a few nights during the week, which exposed an awareness gap between parents and teens.

The National Sleep Foundation 2007 poll – Women and Sleep surveyed women from eighteen to sixty-four years of age and revealed the ongoing state of affairs—persistent sleeplessness and sleep loss. This was the first poll to study women throughout their life cycle, including surveying postpartum women. Approximately 67 percent of respondents reported any sleep problem at least a few nights a week and 46 percent reported difficulty sleeping every night or almost every night. An overwhelming 80 percent admitted to accepting the consequences thereof, such as daytime drowsiness and high stress viewing these consequences as just a part of their lot in life and continued on with their daily lives. Tabulated results revealed that the most commonly reported sleep disturbances were noise, children, and pets.

Another not-so-surprising statistic from this poll was that 72 percent of mothers working outside of the home and 67 percent of single working women complained of insomnia. Snoring and symptoms of sleep apnea or restless legs syndrome were reported by 42 percent of women surveyed.

The following is a brief summary of a few of the highlights from the 2008 through 2011 NSF polls. One should note that many good sleep hygiene tips outlined in this book are supported by the outcomes of these polls:

The National Sleep Foundation 2008 poll—Sleep, Performance, and the Workplace demonstrated a trend that undoubtedly effected work performance. Long work hours (ten or more hours each day) and bringing work home, which translated into extending work hours late into the evening or night, were causing Americans to doze on the job and while driving. Among the poll respondents, 29 percent reported they fell asleep or became very sleepy at work in the past month, and 36 percent reported falling asleep or nodding off while driving in the year prior to the poll. More than 25 percent of respondents reported that they frequently found it difficult to concentrate at work at least a few days a month, a result that may be related to longer workdays and lack of sleep.

The National Sleep Foundation 2009 poll—Health and Safety revealed over the eight previous years an alarming downward trend in the total number of hours of sleep each night. The number of individuals who reported sleeping less than six hours a night had increased, and those who reported sleeping eight hours or more had decreased. In addition, 28 percent of respondents reported driving drowsy at least once in the year prior to taking the poll. Individuals who reported sleeping less than six hours often reported feeling too tired to work efficiently, to exercise, or to prepare and eat healthy meals.

The National Sleep Foundation 2010 poll—Sleep and Ethnicity compared the sleep habits, practices, and attitudes of Asians, African Americans, Hispanics, and Euro-Americans between 25 and 60 years of age. Seventy-one percent of African-Americans reported praying or doing some other religious activity every night prior to bedtime versus 45 percent of Hispanics, 32 percent of Euro-Americans, and 18 percent of Asian-Americans. On average, about 25 percent of all respondents stated that their current work schedule did not allow them to get enough sleep on a daily basis. Although more than 25 percent of respondents on the average assumed that their sleep problems would just go away in time, more than 60 percent on the average stated that they took some action to address their sleep problems. This might indicate that as opposed to earlier polls Americans are becoming ill at ease about lack of sleep.

In 2011, the National Sleep Foundation conducted two polls. The first poll —Technology and Sleep revealed that the vast majority of respondents (95 percent) used some electronic technology, such as a computer, video game, cell phone, or television, within the hour before bedtime on at least a few nights a week. Generational comparison using a standard clinical assessment tool revealed that 20 percent of generation Z'ers (thirteen to eighteen-year-olds) and Y'ers (19 to 29 year-olds) rated themselves as "sleepy", as opposed to only 10 percent of baby boomers (46 to 64 year-olds). Fifty percent of generation Y'ers reported driving drowsy at least once in the month preceding the poll.

The second 2011 poll—Bedroom, uncovered key bedroom elements of respondents age 25-55 years and examined the bedroom environment's effect on sleep. Seventy-one percent of individuals polled reported that they had a television in the bedroom and 11 percent stated they left the television on all night long. Slightly over 90 percent rated a comfortable mattress and pillows important to getting a good night's sleep. Fresh sheets factored in next for 78% of respondents as a favorable incentive to going to bed at night. A surprise to the polltakers was that alarm clocks still factored prominently (89 percent of respondents) in American bedrooms.

Sleep and sleep-related problems can play a significant role in a number of human disorders, and their effects have been seen in almost every field of medicine. It is well-known that problems like stroke and asthma attacks tend to occur more frequently during the night and early morning, which may be due to changes in hormones, heart rate, and other characteristics associated with sleep. Sleep also affects certain forms of epilepsy in complex ways. REM sleep appears to help prevent seizures that start in one section of the brain from spreading to other brain regions, while deep sleep may promote the spread of these seizures.

During a 1998 interview commenting on a historical perspective of sleep, William C. Dement, MD, PhD, of professor emeritus of Stanford University, a pioneer in sleep research who has been studying sleep for more than half a century stated: "Pervasive sleep deprivation and undiagnosed sleep disorders are arguably one of our largest health problems (in America)". Indeed, it is possible that extreme sleep deprivation can lead to a psychotic-like state of paranoia and hallucinations in an otherwise healthy person. Individuals with schizophrenia commonly have sleep disturbances. Acute and chronic exacerbations of schizophrenic episodes are associated with severe insomnia. According to a German research study published in 2014 by Petrovsky and Ettinger et al. prolonged sleep deprivation or severe insomnia can trigger a syndrome that is very similar to paranoid schizophrenia. The researchers demonstrated that after 24 hours of sleep deprivation, healthy individuals displayed symptoms of psychosis similar to those observed in schizophrenia. This research was a proof-of-concept study, which is likely to spawn other validation studies in an effort to demonstrate that a known reliable biomarker of schizophrenia and other schizo-affective disorders is present during prolonged sleep deprivation. Targeting this key biomarker of psychosis triggered by sleep deprivation could have potential importance in research on new antipsychotic drugs.

"My mind clicks on and off. I try letting one eyelid close at a time while I prop the other with my will. But the effect is too much, sleep is winning, my whole body argues dully that nothing, nothing life can attain is quite so desirable as sleep. My mind is losing resolution and control." This was Charles Lindbergh's description of himself nineteen-plus hours into his historic thirty-three-and-a-half-hour May 20, 1927, transatlantic flight from New York to Paris. In his autobiography *The Spirit of St. Louis*, Lindbergh stated that by the time he landed in Paris he had been awake fifty-five hours.

What do you do when your mind just won't turn off and let you sleep? Many people lie awake in bed at night, trying to fall asleep, but their thoughts just keep coming. Below are a few tips to help one get a sweet and more blissful night's sleep. First, if you can't sleep, it is a good idea to take inventory as to why. Ask yourself: Are you running around all day without a minute of real rest and downtime?

Before lying down for the night, the mind needs time to process the day's happenings and get some daytime rest and relaxation (i.e., downtime from the day's activities). Yes, most of the time it is not a good idea to have a working lunch hour. At the end of your workday, make a task list, ranking tasks for the next few days in the order of priority and importance. Always put very important future events or plans down on your calendar as soon as you make them so that you won't forget. You can also put an electronic reminder or alert on your preferred electronic device, which can help to set your mind at ease and allow you to sleep without worrying that you might forget an important date. These end-of-the-day tasks can help you to avoid feeling stressed about all the things that must be done the next day, the next couple of days, or the next week.

Early in the evening, if possible, try to spend some time with family, friends, or other loved ones. Develop and follow an enjoyable routine for winding down at the end of the day. In the few hours before bedtime, straighten things up around the house, especially your bedroom, and prepare for the next day. Make a written priority list of things that need to be done the next day.

If you decide to listen to some music, it should be soft and soothing—not loud or with a fast beat or tempo. You might want to read a chapter or two in a book that you are reading just for pleasure or entertainment.

In at least the one hour before bedtime, there should be no technology use (no television, video games, cell phones, computers—desktops, laptops, or mobile tablets). According to a January 2014 Pew Research Center Report generated from the Center's Internet & American Life Project, interruption of one's sleep throughout the night by a loud ringing cell phone, text alert, or bright computer screen can leave one feeling groggy and sluggish the next day. In addition, being suddenly awakened by midnight e-mails or cell phone calls can lead to mental fatigue. The verification that these kinds of outcomes were indeed possible was supported by two survey research studies investigating the consequences of late-night smartphone use (Lanaj, Johnson, and Barnes 2014). The first study of mid- to high-level managers enrolled in weekend MBA classes indicated that people who monitored their smartphones for business purposes after 9:00 p.m. were more tired, less focused, and less engaged at work the following day. The second study of a more diverse group of US workers compared smartphone usage to other electronic devices and found that smartphones had a larger negative effect than any individual one of the following: watching television, using a laptop or using a mobile electronic tablet.

Solid preparation for the next day can be a real anxiety relief. You won't be thinking in the back of your mind of what you need to do to prepare for the next day when you should instead be relaxing your mind and meditating on peaceful and pleasant thoughts as you drift off to sleep.

Are you constantly worrying about the past and what you or someone else could have said or done differently? If you're trying to understand or relive the past, remember that you cannot undo the past. The past is history; what was done is done. Hopefully you can take the lessons and insight from the past, learn from them, free your mind, and move on. The only time you have is today; tomorrow is not promised to you. Don't waste your today worrying, regretting, and grieving over yesterday. Instead of counting your many mistakes and errors, name your countless blessings! You may find that your cup is not just half-full but may be actually running over!

How about meditating on Psalm 23:

> The Lord is my shepherd, I lack nothing.
> He makes me lie down in green pastures, he leads me beside quiet waters,
> he refreshes my soul. He guides me along the right paths for his name's sake.
> Even though I walk through the darkest valley, I will fear no evil,
> for you are with me; your rod and your staff, they comfort me.
> You prepare a table before me in the presence of my enemies.
> You anoint my head with oil; my cup overflows.
> Surely your goodness and love will follow me all the days of my life,
> and I will dwell in the house of the Lord forever.

Are you mulling over a particular situation in your mind over and over again, trying to figure out the perfect solution or even trying to solve world peace, when you should be sleeping? Remember, whatever the problem or situation you are mulling over in your mind, you cannot develop and implement the best solution in your mind during the middle of the night. To be fresh and ready to go the next day with any ideas that may have come to mind, your best preparation is a good night's sleep. Do not stay up late worrying and thinking about tomorrow's problems and solutions. After a good night's sleep, your thinking will be clearer. When you arise, give yourself plenty of time to get ready for your day, and as you are prepare for the day, prayerfully ask the Lord to guide and assist you throughout the day. If you wish, jot down any thoughts and ideas that come to mind. You will then be more at ease as you face your day—issues and all.

Is the excitement of the next day or near future preventing you from settling down to a restful night's sleep? In the hour or two before you lie down, try to do some mundane activity that will occupy and refocus your mind and let you unwind. Do some light laundry or ironing, or load the dishwasher. Write out a to-do or checklist for your next exciting adventure or fun activity. Post your list where it will be easily accessible, and you will remember where it is when the time comes to get ready for your exciting adventure or fun activity.

Keeping these concerns in mind, I believe that in the primary care setting, obtaining a sleep assessment (paying particular attention to evaluation of sleep habits) should become a standard element on the complete annual history and physical. Health-care providers should be asking their patients about the quality and quantity of their sleep. As stated previously, at least 40 million Americans suffer from sleep disorders, and 20 million more experience occasional sleeping difficulties. According to the NSF's "25 Random Facts about Sleep" more than 60 percent of the time physicians reveal that they do have enough time to discuss sleep during a routine office visit. The standard sleep history should include the following questions: Do you sleep well? If not, then can you tell me why? How long do you sleep? Do you have problems breathing during sleep? Do you experience daytime somnolence (falling asleep when it's important to stay awake)? Have patients list their sleep habits (see sleep health history example—Appendix A).

A number of studies have shown that lack of sufficient sleep stimulates certain hormones that cause sweet and fatty food cravings. A small study at the University of Chicago (Spiegel, Tasali, Penev, and van Cauter 2004) demonstrated that partial sleep deprivation has an immediate effect on altering the circulating levels of ghrelin and leptin, hormones that regulate hunger. Ghrelin is a hormone produced in the stomach that sends out hunger signals to the brain, which then directs an interest in food and stimulates the appetite. Leptin is produced by fat cells and delivers satiation signals to the brain. For this study conducted in the General Clinical Research Center's sleep laboratory at the University of Chicago, a group of twelve healthy young men participated in a 2-part study conducted six weeks apart. Six of the 12 young men randomly selected performed the first part of the study with restricted time in bed and were forced to function on four hours of sleep a night for two nights. The remaining 6 young men first performed the second part of the study but with an extended time of 10 hours in bed. Their appetite-regulating hormone levels and appetite were then measured. Leptin levels were significantly decreased, ghrelin levels were significantly increased and as a result hunger and appetite were also increased. The next year, these researchers performed a crossover study, in which the young men returned to the sleep laboratory, but were allowed a full night's rest and sleep for six nights and repeat measurements were made. On the basis of direct comparison, the men during the sleep-deprived week not only showed statistically significant lower levels of leptin and higher levels of ghrelin, but they also reported an increased appetite especially for high carbohydrate dense foods such as sweet, fatty, starchy and salty foods. The researchers also performed parallel studies on two groups of elderly men with similar results.

Additional findings from the original study in young men revealed that when the study sample was placed on a restricted sleep schedule of four hours each night for six consecutive nights, they showed altered metabolism of glucose, with an insulin resistance pattern similar to that observed in elderly men. Thus, these results revealed a net effect of increasing the subjects' appetite and preference for calorie-dense, high-carbohydrate foods.

Another study in 2004, by Dr. Shahrad Teheri, an endocrinologist at Bristol University, reported a striking connection between the amount of sleep and levels of appetite-regulating hormones in the body. He and his colleagues used data from the Wisconsin Sleep Cohort, an ongoing population-based longitudinal study which began in 1988 and continues to track the sleep habits of over 1,000 volunteers. Teheri and his colleagues' findings suggest that chronic sleep deprivation can lead to individuals becoming overweight or obese. Specifically, they found that people who slept five compared to eight hours each night on the average had a higher body mass index. The CDC defines the body mass index or BMI as a reliable indicator of body fatness for most people, which is useful in screening for weight categories (severely underweight, obese, morbidly obese, or super morbidly obese) that may lead to health problems.

Blood samples from the sleep-deprived volunteers had higher levels of ghrelin, but lower levels of leptin. The researchers concluded that this particular hormonal ratio of high ghrelin/ low leptin was probably encouraging this subgroup of sleep-deprived volunteers to load up on excess calories. Therefore, it is possible to conclude from these studies that there is a strong indication that a few nights of sleep loss can trick your brain into thinking your body needs more food, encouraging you to eat more, placing you at increased risk for obesity. In addition, when we are tired, there is a tendency to try quick pick-me-ups, such as loading up on junk food and drinking coffee.

Too many of us have the head–in-the-sand way of thinking when it comes to establishing good sleep habits. Even in the face of overt chronic signs and symptoms of sleep deprivation, which tell us something is not right with our sleep, we still ignore these warnings. Although a glossary of common sleep disorders is provided in appendix C, you are encouraged to choose a book or two from the bibliography section of this book and read more about the benefits of healthy sleep. In addition, you will find some eye-opening personal stories of healthy normal sleepers who experienced temporary or situational sleep deprivation and sleep debt. You might want to know why I am asking you to read books by other authors. It is because I want those of you who think, "It will never happen to me," to know that for whatever reasons, dire regrettable consequences can and will happen to you when you build up enough sleep debt. So, remember when you incur sleep debt, the only acceptable currency to settle this debt is sleep—payable only in denominations of minutes and hours.

Sleep Loss in the Hospitalized Patient

Okay, we are now getting the picture that sleep is God's medicine. So, why do we ignore this essential therapeutic modality in the majority of acute-care hospitals and skilled nursing facility (SNF) settings in America? What makes the situation worse is that everyone talks about how bad it is, but little has been done to remedy the situation. In fact, looking back over the past several years, noise complaints have consistently topped the list over food complaints. It has become somewhat an accepted cliché to say, "You can't get any rest or sleep in a hospital." So, who are the culprits? Finger-pointing can start by turning to the hospital or SNF environment, comprised of ever-present alarming and humming high-technology equipment, medical devices and the presence of direct-care staff. These culprits often contribute unavoidably and significantly to the noise problem because some sleep disturbance is necessary owing to patients' conditions, which require certain prescribed medical, nursing, or surgical intervention. Yet, paradoxically, often patients' conditions require a greater amount of rest and sleep.

Several state boards of nursing now mandate that nursing staff include pain level as the fifth vital sign (heart rate, respiratory rate, blood pressure, and temperature are the other four) that is assessed whenever a patient's vital signs are taken. Patients who are unable to sleep notice pain more and may increase their requests for pain medication.

However, additional blame can be placed on the physical layout of patient units in older hospitals or skilled nursing facilities. After the age of twenty-one, most people are not accustomed to sleeping in a dormitory or ward-like setting (two or more beds per room). Thankfully, however, most modern hospital facilities these days have opted for single-bed private rooms. This being said, we condone and have come to accept a level of nosocomial and iatrogenic sleep disturbance that is unacceptable. We rationalize it with the above physical environmental and therapeutic interventional requirements. Furthermore, other detractors go frequently unchecked, such as late-night television and around-the-clock or revolving-door visitation. Staff and visitors often engage in loud conversation, which is quite disturbing for most anyone who is trying to get some rest or sleep. Finally, unfortunate disturbances also arise from events in the hospital, such as codes, drills, patient outbursts, and open expressions of patient distress.

In 2005, researchers at Johns Hopkins University (Busch-Vishnica, Ilene, West, Barnhill, Hunter, Orellana & Chivukula) began studies investigating the hospital noise problem.

Conclusions drawn from these studies determined that excessive noise not only hindered the ability for patients to obtain much-needed rest, but also raised the risk for medical errors.

Most discussions and studies of noise levels reference an A-weighted sound scale using the unit of decibels (dB). Past clinical studies have demonstrated that throughout the day and night, hospital sound levels in patient-care areas can average greater than 50 dB(A), with transient peaks reaching on the average from 80dB(A) to greater than 100 dB(A). To put these dB sound levels in perspective, below is a comparison list of common sounds and their noise levels measured in dB:

> public one-on-one conversation averages 60dB.
> moderate street traffic noise: approximately 70dB.
> heavy truck moving in traffic: approximately 79dB.
> operation of a chainsaw: approximately 82 dB (comparable to being three feet away from some food processors).
> passing subway train: 100 dB.
> operation of a jackhammer (or a large motorcycle!): approximately 102 dB.
> car horn: approximately 102 dB.
> thunderclap: approximately 130 dB.

Several decades ago the United States Environmental Protection Agency (EPA) provided noise guidelines for hospitals that included a limitation on noise level not to exceed 45 dB during the day. In 1995 the World Health Organization (WHO) established its first guidelines on hospital noise levels. In 1999 the guidelines were updated and published on its website. These guidelines included the recommendation that the equivalent sound pressure level in most rooms where patients reside and are being treated should not exceed 35 dB at any given time with particular attention given to special care areas such as intensive care units. Noise levels in excess of the WHO and EPA guidelines are believed to disturb sleep, contribute to stress, lead to poor recovery from illness, contribute to medication and other care error, and interfere with all forms of communication within the hospital.

Florence Nightingale wrote in her most influential book *Notes on Nursing: What It Is and What It Is Not* (1860, pp. 44, 45-46): "Unnecessary noise, or noise that creates an expectation in the mind, is that which hurts a patient." "... Unnecessary noise, then is the most cruel absence of care which can be inflicted either on sick or well."

Tips on how to address health-care facility noise problems might include:

- Elimination of unnecessary lighting and loud staff conversation, as well as the reduction of necessary lighting levels whenever possible (new and preexisting hospital construction is now including light fixtures with dimmer switches).
- Negotiation (among nurse, doctor, and patient) in terms of time of day and frequency of certain patient interventions, such as vital signs and noncritical blood draws and other routine procedures.
- Maintenance of adequate pain-relief measures during hospitalization: encourage routine and as-needed pain medication to avoid getting behind on pain control; assist with positioning while lying in bed or when sitting up in a chair; remember to offer pain medication before activities that might induce pain.
- Minimization of the amount of in-hospital room equipment that beeps or alarms. This may be costly to the hospital, but there is developing technology where

these alerts are placed just outside the patient's room or at the nursing station.

- Guarding against patient fatigue by spacing all activities with adequate rest periods as needed or requested by patient.

Additional tips on how to address hospital noise (Moore, Nolan, Nguyen & Ryals, et al. 1998) (Yoder, 2012) might include:

- Better adherence to established visiting hours. It is reasonable and compassionate to accommodate important visitors, such as family, close friends, and the clergy, because of their work schedule and other demands that preclude them from observing regular visiting hours;
- However, all visitors should at all times respect the dignity and quietude of the hospital environment (which means before entering a shared room, first gently knock; and which may involve checking in at the nursing station before proceeding to a patient's room, respecting the privacy of all patients encountered, and not engaging in loud conversation or laughter).
- Better management of sleeping problems in patients who have other medical/surgical conditions. This will definitely improve their health and quality of life.

Please do not be dismayed by all that has been mentioned above in this chapter. All is not lost; there is good news: a growing number of hospitals are working toward a new era of quiet. There are programs such as "Quiet Hospital," in which there are posters and staff who sport badges with this motto on them. Other facilities have instituted "Quiet at Night" campaigns (from 9:00 p.m. to 6:00 a.m.), with this slogan posted at the entrance on every unit and unit "Quiet Champions" who encourage and support staff in the use of noise-reduction strategies (Murphy, Bernardo, Dalton, 2013).

"The hospital is not a hotel!" Sound familiar? In point of fact, hotels are part of the "hospital"-ity industry, so where is the hospitable part in our hospitals today? Many models of hospital-based care operate on the premise that patients have to fairly rigidly follow the hospital's set routines, schedules, and disease-specific protocols, and they must accept only the choice of goods and services offered in their hospital.

In 2001, the Institute of Medicine (IOM) issued a report with the following recommendations: health-care delivery systems are strongly advised to become patient-centered, rather than clinician- or disease-centered, with treatment recommendations and decision making customized to patients 'needs, preferences and values. One of the aspects of the IOM's patient-centered model is that care is based upon continuous healing relationships and environments. This model includes the requirement that health-care delivery systems provide for the physical comfort and emotional support of patients and their families.

CHAPTER 7

---◈---

Holistic Benefits of Sleep

Why is it so important to acknowledge and understand that sleep is a therapeutic gift from God?

The benefits of sleep—oh, let me count the ways …

The benefits of obtaining an optimum daily amount of sleep and the serious negative consequences of chronic sleep deprivation are probably some of the best clinical evidence of the mind-body-spirit connection. Evidence of the true therapeutic interaction of these three aspects of our total being is found in their association or linkage during sleep. It is precisely this interplay that allows us to rise each day as fully functioning and well-balanced healthy individuals. For most adults an optimum daily amount of sleep means getting approximately eight hours of sleep each night.

During these times of high stress-filled living, pollution, and chronic immune system attack, the therapeutic benefits of a good night's sleep help keep us in balance. If your very being is now connecting and responding to something you have read thus far—and you hear, listen, and act—you are gaining very important knowledge and understanding right now.

There is a deep everlasting spiritual connection and love between God and man that is manifested through His boundless blessings and gifts. He always knows what we need and supplies all that we need through His riches and glory in Christ Jesus. Loving God and receiving God's blessings and love spiritually renews us. There is an interconnection between experiencing good sleep on a daily basis and maintaining good spiritual sleep habits. One provides the energy and healthy mind-set to devote oneself in turn to the other. When considering sleep and spiritual blessings, we realize that we can strengthen our connection to Him through practicing good spiritual sleep habits, including praying, listening to relaxing and inspiring holy music, and reading and meditating on God's Word.

Also, as just mentioned above, there is a connection between the gifts of God and our well-being. The nightly partaking of God's therapeutic gift of sleep allows us to attain tremendous spiritual, mental, and physical benefits. Making sure that one routinely obtains good sleep, both in quantity and quality, promotes good health and wholeness through actively enabling the innate connections among our mind, body, and spirit to function for our benefit. We show our appreciation for His gifts by accepting and using them always for His glory and honor, that is, by accepting them for the express purpose for which they were given, our personal benefit and well-being as well as those of others. Getting sufficient sleep is necessary for a healthy body, a healthy mind, and a right spirit. All of this prepares us for daily service to God, family, and community.

> "Therefore, I urge you, brothers and sisters, in view of God's mercy, to offer your bodies as a living sacrifice, holy and pleasing to God—this is your true and proper worship. Do not conform to the pattern of this world, but be transformed by the renewing of your mind. Then you will be able to test and

approve what God's will is—his good, pleasing and perfect will." (Rom. 12:1–2)

In this passage the apostle Paul conveys the message that we are not only to present our physical bodies to God, but also our minds, hearts, and spirit—our entire being. A person's body, mind, spirit, and heart all matter to God. As followers of Christ, we belong to Him body and soul. In Him our bodies have been made alive from spiritual death and sanctified to His service. Our bodies are holy, separated from the world, reserved for God's use alone and His eternal purposes.

The presenting or offering of our bodies involves our bodily behavior. In presenting our bodies as a living sacrifice, it is this living that is our act of worship "…holy, acceptable to God, which is your reasonable service" (Romans 12:1, KJV). This passage describes an act of worship, and God is the center of that worship. In terms of sleep, an appreciative attitude or mind toward sleep and the act of obtaining proper sleep are (as are all our acts of daily living) part of our worship toward God. Having an appreciative attitude or mind toward sleep is embodied in "…renewing your mind" (Romans 12:2, KJV) and is obtained by being saturated in the Word of God. This means each day we are to read, study, and meditate on His Word. The exact time you spend on each of these acts is entirely up to you. It is important that you engage in all three on a daily basis. In addition, all God's people should develop the spiritual practice of daily prayer and devotion. In this manner we learn to love the Lord our God with all our heart, all our life, all our strength, and with all our mind.

We are to glorify and honor the Lord in our bodies. For believers in Christ, bodies are the temples of God, in which the Holy Spirit dwells.

"Do you not know that your bodies are temples of the Holy Spirit, who is in you, whom you have received from God? You are not your own; you were bought at a price. Therefore honor God in your bodies." (1 Cor. 6:19–20).

Why Do We Dream When We Sleep?

Dreaming and sleep are integrally related. One of the primary reasons we need to sleep is precisely so that we may dream. It is scientifically proven that deep sleep is associated with dreaming. The Bible further defines deep sleep: it is the state in which dreams and visions occur. Scripture also defines stages of sleep: deep sleep and slumber. Slumber is light sleep.

God provided a deep sleep for Abraham to show him the prophecy of his descendants taken into captivity as slaves in Egypt for four hundred years (Gen. 15:12).

Jacob was asleep on "pillow stones" when he was given his vision about the ladder up into heaven (Gen. 28:11–16).

In 1 Samuel 26:12, God caused a deep sleep to fall upon Saul and his men, so that David would know he could trust Him for protection from his enemies.

Job's friend Eliphaz in Job 4:12–13 tells of his revealing vision in the night that spoke of how God's judgments (unto eternal condemnation) are not for the righteous and that to err is part of the human condition: "Now a thing was secretly brought to me, and mine ear received a whisper of it. In disquieting thoughts from the visions of the night, when deep sleep falls on men … " Later on in Job 33:14–18, the prophet Elihu offers Job reason for sleep, informing him that God calls men to repentance by visions.

For God may speak in one way or another, yet man does not perceive it. In a dream, in a vision of the night, when deep sleep falls upon men, while slumbering upon their beds, Then He opens the ears of men, and seals their instruction. In order to turn man from his deed, And conceal pride from man, He keeps back his soul from the Pit, and his life from perishing by the sword.

Samuel while sleeping received his preordained calling from God (1 Sam. 3:1–10).

The transfiguration vision was given after three disciples were asleep (Luke 9:32, Matt. 17:1–9).

The language of dreams is partly symbolic. Symbolism is the primary means by which many spiritual thoughts, perspectives, and attitudes are presented to our consciousness. Dream symbols cannot be standardized; they are highly individualized. The ancient Israelites had one word for both "to dream" and "to see."

God appeared to King Solomon at night in a dream to bestow on him blessings like no other earthly king had ever (or would ever) receive.

Then God said to him: "Because you have asked this thing, and have not asked for long life for yourself, ... but have asked for yourself understanding to discern justice, behold, I have done according to your words; see, I have given you a wise and understanding heart, so that there has not been anyone like you before you, nor shall any like you arise after you ... And I have also given you what you have not asked: both riches and honor, so that there shall not be anyone like you among the kings all your days. So if you walk in My ways, to keep My statutes and My commandments, as your father David walked, then I will lengthen your days. (1 Kings 3:11–14 NKJV)

King Nebuchadnezzar of Babylon couldn't sleep because his dreams troubled him and he couldn't understand them (Dan. 2:1). God caused these dreams and revealed their meaning to Daniel to inform the king and for our understanding of His works in the Old Testament. Daniel had prophetic visions while in a deep sleep (Dan. 8:18, 10:9).

The angel of the LORD revealed the truth about Mary's conception to Joseph in a dream (Matt. 1:18–25).

From the above Bible passages, we see that God sometimes communicated His message to people during their sleep or caused a deep sleep to overtake a person to accomplish His purpose. Therefore, spiritually we can believe that God causes deep sleep and dreaming that occurs during this stage for an informing purpose, one from which we can gain wisdom and insight. This is perhaps why the advice to "sleep on it" may not be such a bad idea when faced with a difficult decision or problem. Mentally, dreaming allows us to subconsciously solve problems and to use what we have learned when we awaken. What can be postulated from these biblical passages is that God spoke to Old Testament prophets and individuals during sleep and particularly during dream sleep when willful individual human thought processes are less likely to intervene, long-term emotional memory tracks are produced, and one is able to create mental images and recognize familiar and unfamiliar faces. Scientifically this divine purpose is supported by the following anatomical facts:

- The limbic system is considered the brain's long-term emotional center. During REM sleep and dreaming, the amygdala, a structural part of the limbic system of the brain, is highly active. The amygdala is an important structure in memory, particularly long-term emotional memory.

- During sleep, the visual association area (the area of the brain that is involved in creating mental images and recognizing faces) is active above waking levels.

- Recent research has linked motivation, goal seeking, and problem solving with the ability to dream. These functions may lie at the basis of naturally occurring lucid dreaming. Lucid dreams are most often fleeting experiences that occur just before awakening. As stated previously lucid dreamers are consciously aware of dreaming in the midst of a dream. Sometimes the dreamer successfully directs or controls his or her actions. Often the lucid dreamer can also successfully direct or control the actions of others while dreaming. Occasionally I have awakened from a lucid dream feeling slightly frustrated because I awoke before completing the direction of my dream scenario. In the quiet of the night, psychologically I reassure myself that this outcome was all right because it was just a dream. Lucid dreaming only occurs during REM sleep, a highly metabolically active sleep state.

A word of caution is due: God's prophecy to humanity has been fulfilled in His Son, Jesus Christ. Therefore, today when we dream, God is not revealing His prophecy to us. Yet God is still speaking to us. We should not venture to substitute dreams and dream symbols for the spiritual direction and guidance we receive from the Holy Spirit, through personal prayer, meditation, and fasting—and of course, reading and studying the Bible.

Joseph of the Bible says that dreams belong to God and He does not want us to look at the past (Gen. 40:8). This means God wants us to be in the present and look forward to the glorious future He has in store for us. Luke 12:11-12 states "...do not worry about how you will defend yourselves or what you will say, for the Holy Spirit will teach you at that time what you should say."

"But the Helper, the Holy Spirit, whom the Father will send in my name, He will teach you all things and bring to your remembrance all that I have said to you. Peace I leave with you, My peace I give to you; not as the world gives do I give to you. Let not your heart be troubled, neither let it be afraid" (John 14:26–27).

Furthermore in 1 Cor. 2:9-11 we find the following passage:

> However, as it is written:
> "What no eye has seen, what no ear has heard, and what no human mind has conceived"— the things God has prepared for those who love him—these are the things God has revealed to us by his Spirit.
>
> The Spirit searches all things, even the deep things of God. For who knows a person's thoughts except their own spirit within them? In the same way no one knows the thoughts of God except the Spirit of God.

Most of a night's sleep is spent in deep sleep, when new growth and cell and tissue repair occur. Some research experts believe neurons that are active when we are awake are given the chance to shut down for self-repair while we are asleep. Without sleep our neurons may become so energy-depleted or so polluted with the by-products of normal cellular activities that they eventually begin to malfunction. Sleep may also give the brain the opportunity to exhibit important neuronal connections that would otherwise run a high risk of deterioration from a lack of activity.

REM sleep stimulates brain regions used in learning. Past preliminary human and animal studies suggested that REM sleep in early infancy provides nerve stimulation that aids in visual cortex development and assists in the programming of developing neuronal circuits (Marks, Shaffery and Roffwarg, 1995, 1999; Frank, Issa, and Stryker et al., 2001). These findings indicate a very important role for REM sleep in normal brain development during the neonatal period and in early infancy. In addition, this may be the reason why infants spend significantly more time in REM sleep than do adults.

Memory and sleep, particularly REM sleep, are integrally related. In fact, proper sleep actually improves memory. REM sleep facilitates learning and memory through the organization and consolidation of long-term memories and daily brain-function renewal. As a part of learning, sleep allows the mind to acquire new tasks by mixing short- and long-term memories while we sleep, reinforcing what we have learned during the day.

Control of our emotional responses and the ability to exercise appropriate decision making are healthy benefits of good sleep hygiene, that is, good sleep habits. Sleep allows the body to rest and the mind to sort out past, present, and future activities and feelings. A small comparison study at Rush-Presbyterian St. Luke's Medical Center in Chicago, Illinois suggested that the more REM sleep we get, the more likely we are to wake up in a good mood feeling positive and upbeat (Cartwright, Luten, Young, Mercer, & Bears, 1998). Their findings supported other studies that found a positive relationship between REM sleep and emotional relaxation and REM sleep and rejuvenation.

Proper sleep helps judgment, reaction time (which involves our neuroreflexes and hand-eye coordination), and daytime alertness and improves motor (physical) activity. During sleep the brain performs vital housekeeping tasks, such as integrating new information, providing for the repair and renewal of tissue and nerve cells, and replenishing certain neuroactive molecules.

Therefore, one would be correct to assert that sleeping is probably our most valuable physical activity of the day. Sleep is not wasted or empty time spent doing nothing. It allows us to maximize the time and energy that we expend throughout the day. Waking up from a good night's sleep is both refreshing and actually "feels sweet."

Historically, the subject of proper sleep during medical school and residency training was given no more than a respectful nod as being important to the maintenance of good physical, mental and emotional health. However, with the growth and advancements in sleep medicine and research over the past few decades, this situation has been slowing changing. Furthermore, we are seeing an increase in the discipline of integrative medicine being added to the curriculum in medical schools and specialty training across the United States. In the not-too-distant future, I hope a course in "Holistic Sleep" will be part of the regular curricula in undergraduate, graduate, and professional schools across the country.

Sleep is one of those life-sustaining essentials that, when adequate daily amounts are obtained, enable us to fully express the "fruit of the Spirit" in our life, which according to Galatians 5:22 are love, joy, peace, patience, kindness, goodness, faithfulness, gentleness, and self-control. Have you ever seen a chronically sleep-deprived person exercise much patience and self-control?

Nursing school students are taught "The Five Rights to Medication Administration" (actually there are six because complete and accurate documentation is also considered a right or a must). These same rights apply when we view sleep as God's medicine and are as follows:

The Right Drug—Sleep is an essential biological function necessary for human life itself; there are no viable substitutes.

The Right Patient—All human beings require sleep.

The Right Dose— Proper functioning on a daily basis requires an optimum amount of sleep; too little or too much can have adverse "drug" effects.

The Right Time—Humans are diurnal, not nocturnal, beings; we are divinely designed to be awake in the daytime and to sleep at night.

The Right Route—The lying-down position is not only the most comfortable for sleeping, but also bodily activities that must occur during sleep function better in the fully reclined position.

When sleep does not come naturally as God planned it, there are a number of things that one can do to correct this problem. Acknowledging and following the above rights of sleep-medication administration can help us obtain the quantity and quality of sleep we need each night. Use them to gain helpful insight into the principles and practice of good sleep hygiene (i.e. daily habits and practices beneficial to obtaining restful sleep), the topic of our next two chapters.

CHAPTER 8

Principles of Good Sleep Hygiene or Sleep Premedication

The establishment of good sleep hygiene or sleep habits is to the healthy functioning body what Florence Nightingale's introduction of good hand washing (basic hygiene) and other simple sanitation measures were to the soldiers in the Crimean War—indispensable and lifesaving. Good sleep habits, once established, can lead to a remarkable improvement in one's overall health and well-being. In addition, one can expect to experience significant improvement in one's ability to function and adapt to internal and external stressors.

The basics of good sleep hygiene or habits are what I call premedication for sleep. Sleep premedication is analogous to what is provided in real-life hospital settings or clinical practice. Certain premedications, such as a sedative-hypnotic (Midazolam—Versed®), anxiolytic (Xanax®, Ativan®), or analgesic (morphine or hydromorphone—Dilaudid®) medications are used to prepare and relax patients before the administration of general anesthesia and the start of surgery or other medical-surgical procedures requiring conscious sedation. Other premedications are given for the purpose of induction (the facilitation of the administration of anesthesia or the beginning of stage 1 of general anesthesia). The establishment of good sleep hygiene (i.e., habits) prepares one for sleep.

How does one establish good sleep habits? It is important to maintain regular exposure to daylight throughout the week so that your body recognizes night from day. If you work indoors, try to take at least one break outside in the sunlight. If you work at night, try to obtain a couple of hours of actual daylight during the day.

Don't go to bed unless you are sleepy and ready to sleep. If you are not sleepy at bedtime, stay up or get up and find something else to do that will take your mind off of worrying about not being able to sleep. Choose a relaxing lightweight activity to distract your mind so you won't continue to worry about not being able to sleep. Pray especially if you feel the need, take a warm soaking bath, read a few minutes of a non-action packed book, or listen to soft quiet music. In addition, you might try relaxation techniques, such as performing deep breathing exercises, motion exercises such as Tai Chi, or meditation.

Since melatonin is produced mainly at night (and known to induce sleep), in 1995 researchers (Massion, Teas, Hebert, Wertheimer, and Jon Kabat-Zinn) at the University of Massachusetts Medical Center's Mindfulness-Based Stress Reduction Program, conducted a study measuring 6-sulphatoxymelatonin, a melatonin breakdown product excreted in the urine at night which is thought to be an accurate reflection of blood melatonin levels. The researchers found that women who regularly meditated had significantly higher levels of this breakdown product compared with women who did not meditate.

After going to bed, if you are not asleep after twenty minutes, get out of bed. Follow the same advice for relaxation above. If you can, do this in another room. The bed is not a place to go when you are bored. Once you feel sleepy again, go back to bed.

Develop and maintain evening rituals that help you relax and feel at ease before bedtime. Create a routine that prepares you for sleep. Your practice could include some of the relaxation exercises or techniques mentioned above. Many studies have shown that people who routinely practice evening rituals in preparation for going to bed sleep better. A warm relaxing bath just before bedtime will help because afterward, as one's moist skin dries, the body cools down, and this cooling induces sleep. Some individuals have found that a small glass of milk routinely taken about an hour before bedtime helps them to fall asleep. Milk can also help to deepen one's level of sleep.

Rise at the same time every morning, including weekends and holidays. This helps one maintain a good sleep-wake routine and improves daytime functioning and efficiency. Avoid the tendency to sleep in later on the weekends to catch up on lost sleep.

Strive for a full night's sleep on a consistent regular basis. Plan to go to bed early enough so that you will have seven to eight hours before you have to get up in the morning. Set it as a goal and make it a priority. Keep a sleep diary of your daily waking and sleeping schedule that can help you determine your most restful sleep period. A sleep diary can also assist your primary care provider in assessing your sleeping difficulties by evaluating the frequency and intensity of your sleep arousals and your difficulty in falling or staying asleep. An example of a sleep diary is in Appendix B.

Try to sleep through the night by minimizing wake-ups during the night. Many studies have shown that sleep is most restful and restorative when it is relatively continuous without periodic waking. Avoid drinking water just before going to bed, which helps prevent nocturia or nighttime waking to urinate.

In the morning when you wake up, get out of bed and stay up. Don't linger in bed trying to snooze after you wake up. Get out of bed and expose yourself to natural sunlight as soon as you can.

Although naps can be restorative, avoid taking naps if you can. If you must take a nap, try to keep it short (not more than a half hour) and take it in the early afternoon at the optimum time of between 1:00 p.m. and 3:00 p.m., which coincides with your second naturally occurring circadian-rhythm sleep drive. Napping after 3:00 p.m., especially long napping, can make it more difficult to fall asleep at night. For most people naps, especially in the evening, disrupt the normal sleep-wake cycle and are not beneficial to a good night's sleep. For some a short mild exercise or stretching routine may be more beneficial than a nap to promote a good night's sleep.

Keep a regular daily routine or schedule. This means maintaining regular times for meals, medications, housework, exercise, and other activities. In other words a daily routine helps you to stay in tune with your body's natural circadian rhythm and to keep it running smoothly.

Reserve the bed only for sleeping or intimacy. Don't read, write, eat, watch television, talk on the phone, or play cards in bed. Although many people can fall asleep while watching television, the light from the screen can still cause one to have a less-than-restful sleep.

De-clutter your bedroom. Mental and physical clutter help define the least-conducive environment for sleep. Make sure you can tell your bedroom from your attic. Resist making your bedroom a multipurpose room—your mini-storage, home office, leisure-activities room, and second wet bar. Airflow is improved in an uncluttered environment, and therefore breathing and thus sleeping are also better in an uncluttered bedroom.

Turn your bedroom into a sleep sanctuary. Your décor should reflect an oasis of calm and serenity. Paint your bedroom walls in soothing colors that inspire feelings compatible with rest, relaxation, and sleep—pale blue is very special because it signifies peace, healing, tranquility, joy, spirituality, and sleep; pale yellow is associated with air, symbolizing health, blessing, and creativity; pale pink represents harmony, friendship or friendliness, and affection; medium light green represents restfulness and well-being. Hang paintings that are tranquil and serene. Decorate your bedroom with items that make you feel peaceful, happy, and relaxed. Pictures should be associated with and evoke fond memories and feelings of happiness. Use subdued lighting or lamps.

Choose a bed that is most suitable for you. Choose a bed that is comfortable for you (and your bedmate). Select the bedding (e.g., blankets, pillow, quilt, spreads, duvets) and the mattress that make you feel the most comfortable when you lie down and go to sleep. Consider your bed and bedding as appropriate and necessary durable medical equipment for sleep.

Over ten years ago, most of the major hotel chains decided to make a large investment in their businesses by renovating their guest rooms with signature comfortable beds and bedding. This improvement greatly enhanced the sleep of thousands of travel-weary and sleep-deprived hotel guests all over the world. Subsequently, while attending conferences or conventions, I met several people who shared their experiences with sleeping in these upgraded hotel beds. They did not realize that their bed at home was preventing them from getting a good night's sleep. A comfortable bed can serve to remind us of the overall comfort of home.

For individuals who suffer from environmental insomnia (a condition wherein individuals frequently have a difficult time sleeping in an unfamiliar environment), sometimes bringing along a little bit of home may just do the trick. It might be just the thing that helps—either cuddling up with your favorite throw or pillow, sipping on your hard-to-find-on-the-road favorite herbal tea or other beverage or slipping into your favorite house slippers at bedtime.

Reserve your bed for humans. Furnish your family pet with his or her own little bed next to yours if he or she sleeps in the same room with you.

Turn off the computer at least one hour before bedtime because sitting in front of a light source just before bedtime may affect the biological clock in one's brain and delay the onset of sleep.

Try to fit in physical activity every day, but as much as possible, avoid any vigorous cardiac workout or similar type of exercise within five hours of your bedtime. Studies have shown that better sleep patterns are attained when routine exercise is performed in the late afternoon. The body temperature decreases about five to six hours after late-afternoon exercising, which in turn helps to induce sleep. Afternoon exercising is associated with higher levels of restorative deep stage 3 and 4 sleep. Regular routine exercise itself is associated with taking a shorter time to fall asleep. Avoiding vigorous exercise within five hours of bedtime is important because this form of exercise increases metabolism and levels of the stress hormone cortisol, which can keep you revved up instead of winding down for sleep.

Dietary issues can contribute to insomnia. By making some changes in one's diet or lifestyle, you may be able to improve your quality and quantity of sleep.

Don't eat a big meal near bedtime, and yet do not go to bed hungry either. If hunger associated with an empty stomach keeps you from sleeping, try a very light snack, such as crackers or a piece of fruit before bedtime. Exercise caution not to consume your snack with a large drink, as this in and of itself could cause more nighttime awakenings for bathroom runs. A large meal just before bedtime causes an increase in gastrointestinal blood flow and body temperature for digestion. This event, in turn, can delay the body temperature decrease that helps in sleep induction.

Avoid heavy or spicy foods just prior to bedtime. These meals can interfere with sleep by causing heartburn or aggravate conditions such as hiatal hernia or gastroesophageal reflux disease, commonly known as GERD.

Do not drink any caffeine-containing beverages after lunch because the half-life of caffeine is approximately six hours. The half-life of a drug is the time that it takes 50 percent of the medication to be absorbed, metabolized, and eliminated from the body. Caffeine blocks the neuroreceptors for adenosine, a chemical substance that increases during the day that promotes sleep. Dietary sources of caffeine include coffee, black tea, energy drinks or energy bars, chocolate, many regular soda drinks, and certain foods and medications. Because of this widespread availability of hidden dietary sources of caffeine, it is a good idea to become a label-reader.

Do not have a beer, a glass of wine, or any other alcohol within five hours of your bedtime. Alcohol is the most common sleep medication used in the United States. Alcohol is both a central nervous system stimulant and depressant, depending on the blood levels and time after ingestion. At low levels (one to two drinks), it increases electrical activity in the brain, affecting pleasure and euphoria, easing anxiety, and reducing depression, thus also inducing sleep. Yet in larger amounts, alcohol interferes with messages in the brain; besides making one clumsy and uncoordinated and having a tendency toward slurred speech, it reduces one's ability to learn and form memories. Alcohol consumed at bedtime can exacerbate sleep apnea.

Alcohol intake at both levels can inhibit restful sleep. During the night alcohol can drastically disrupt sleep cycles, thereby reducing sleep efficiency, and can cause rebound excitability. As the body metabolizes alcohol, one is more likely to have frequent awakenings. Alcohol relaxes the throat muscles. When these muscles relax, the throat closes up, making it difficult to breathe, and can cause a person to wake up repeatedly during the night. Collectively, all these factors lead to a non-restful night's sleep. Movement sleep disorders, such as restless legs syndrome and periodic limb movements, can be worsened by the effects of alcohol. It can have a negative effect on the timing of sleep due to interference with melatonin, growth hormone, and serotonin. Alcohol suppresses REM sleep, the stage of sleep during which most dreaming occurs. In addition, it can cause or contribute to problems with snoring. Alcohol is also a diuretic, which can lead to nocturnal bathroom visits. Finally, that bedtime nightcap may cause morning headaches, especially migraine headaches in women who are prone to them.

Do not have a cigarette or any other source of nicotine before bedtime. Nicotine is a central nervouse system (CNS) stimulant; therefore when smokers sleep, they experience a powerful nicotine withdrawal syndrome that produces fast brain-wave activity, promoting frequent episodes of wakefulness. Nicotine causes problems for both falling asleep and waking up. Some studies have shown that smoking is associated with increased nightmares, which of course can disrupt sleep. As you already know, it would be better if you did not use nicotine at all, but if you do, try not to partake within four hours of your bedtime.

Use prescription or over-the-counter sleeping pills with extreme caution and on a limited-time basis (not more than two consecutive weeks) and always under the care of your primary health care provider in order to avoid prolonged dependence on sleep aids. In addition, do not drink alcohol while taking sleeping pills. The interaction can lead to an additive effect with a high potential for serious oversedation.

Use your waking hours to try to get rid of or deal with things that worry you. Avoid worrying about problems at night; instead, try thinking about them during the daytime. The bed is a place for sleep, not a place for anxiety and worry. Don't keep vigil over what time it is getting to be when you should be sleeping; put your clock out of sight during the night. Use your bedtime ritual or routine to distract you from your daily concerns and worries. Worry makes a poor bedfellow. I have a saying: Remember, Mr. Regret and Mr. Worry will never send you back a note saying, "You're welcome; I'm glad I could help you." This does not mean there aren't times for alarm and concern, but we are not to allow ourselves to slip into a state of constant worry or fear.

Since worrying is a big problem in today's society, do not skip over the passages below on why we should not worry:

> "Therefore I say to you, do not worry about your life, what you will eat or what you will drink; nor about your body, what

you will put on. Is not life more than food and the body more than clothing? Look at the birds of the air, for they neither sow nor reap nor gather into barns; yet your heavenly Father feeds them. Are you not of more value than they?" (Matt. 6:25–26 NKJV)

"So why do you worry about clothing? Consider the lilies of the field, how they grow: they neither toil nor spin; and yet I say to you that even Solomon in all his glory was not arrayed like one of these. Now if God so clothes the grass of the field, which today is, and tomorrow is thrown into the oven, will He not much more clothe you, O you of little faith?" (Matt. 6:28–30 NKJV)

"Therefore do not worry, saying, 'What shall we eat?' or 'What shall we drink?' or 'What shall we wear?' For after all these things the [non-believers] seek. For your heavenly Father knows that you need all these things. But seek first the kingdom of God and His righteousness, and all these things shall be added to you. Therefore do not worry about tomorrow, for tomorrow will worry about its own things. Sufficient for the day *is* its own trouble…" (Matthew 6:31–34 NKJV)

"…know that the Lord does not save with sword and spear; for the battle is the Lord's …" (1 Samuel 17:47 NKJV)

"And do not seek what you should eat or what you should drink, nor have an anxious mind. For all these things the nations of the world seek after, and your Father knows that you need these things. But seek the kingdom of God, and all these things shall be added to you…" (Luke 12:29–31 NKJV)

God's desire for every human being is expressed by the author of 3 John 1:2, a leader of a local church, Gaius, who wrote to his friend: "Beloved, I pray that you may prosper in all things and be in health, just as your soul prospers" (NKJV).

It is important to feel safe and secure where you sleep. Therefore if it makes you feel better, then by all means make those nighttime room rounds, door and window lock checks, and whatever else makes you feel comfortable, secure, and ready for bed.

Travelers frequently suffering from jet lag often have the unhealthy habit of worrying about their jet lag. This can make jet lag and temporary insomnia even worse. Remembering the adage that an ounce of prevention is worth a pound of cure, long-distance travelers should plan, and plan ahead of time. Attend to as many business and other personal affairs as possible before the start of a trip in order to avoid any negative consequences that may result from taking that trip for business or pleasure. If you arrive at your destination and it is still daylight, try to expose yourself to the bright sunlight or some other bright artificial light. This will signal your SCN to reset your internal biological clock. Most of us can reset our internal clocks by one or two hours a day. Former US President Nixon often used this strategy when traveling across multiple time zones.

Maintain a quiet, dark, and slightly cool bedroom. Bats are world-class champion sleepers. They normally sleep about sixteen hours each day. Maybe it's because they sleep in dark, cool, and generally quiet caves! Most individuals sleep best in some degree of silence or with monotonous white noise that screens out loud or abrupt and interrupting sounds. The bedroom should be kept as dark as possible, without night-lights or other room lights while sleeping. Many individuals have found that bedroom clock-radios with glow-in-the-dark LCD displays actually cause their eyes to burn or feel irritated. If need be, install light-blocking window coverings. Some may find the use of eyeshades or masks helpful. Warm ambient room temperature usually interrupts sleep. For most people a comfortable temperature for sleeping is around 70 degrees Fahrenheit (I know some like it hot and some like it cold, but many people don't realize that these preferences may be contributing to their restlessness or stirring about during the night). In addition, keep your home dim and quiet in the few hours before bedtime. As the day turns into evening, begin turning down lights and closing window coverings to prevent light from filtering in from the street. This helps to decrease retinal stimulation from light, which cues the brain to awaken us.

If you literally tend to have cold feet, then wear socks to bed. Your feet often feel cold before the rest of the body due to their very peripheral location. Cold feet sometimes can be related to advancing age or disease which can cause poor circulation. Keeping your feet comfortably warm may induce restful sleep and reduce night awakenings.

Seek needed medical attention for any sleep disorder or other sleep-related medical or psychological problems you might have. Treatable conditions include thyroid or cardiovascular disease; respiratory problems such as COPD, sleep apnea, bronchitis, and asthma; urinary problems such as nocturia; gastroesophageal reflux disease (GERD); musculoskeletal disorders such as arthritis or gout; neurological disorders such as restless legs syndrome; and finally, psychiatric disorders such as depression and anxiety.

Two conditions deserve special consideration for discussion: respiratory allergies and GERD. These two are the most notorious sleep robbers ever encountered. Allergies can interfere with sleep due to coughing, nasal congestion, post-nasal drip, or sinus pressure. GERD can cause angina, persistent dry cough, and poor sleep, with distressful wakening from sleep.

There are additional sleep-promoting tips to help respiratory allergy sufferers. Measures that can be taken include:

- Use zippered, allergen-proof covers on all your pillows, mattress, box spring, and other bedding (mattress pad, blanket, duvet, etc.). The zipper and any small opening near the zipper can be covered with fabric-reinforced tape.
- Wash all bedding in hot water if care instructions allow. Studies have shown that 130 degrees Fahrenheit water kills 100 percent of dust mites, but even cold water still kills approximately 90 percent of dust mites.
- Change all bedding once a week, pillow covers every couple of days.
- Keep your hair clean because during the day, dust and pollens cling to the hair shaft, and when you lie down, enough of these allergens are transferred to your pillow to enhance your allergy symptoms.
- Keep the humidity in your bedroom to less than 50 percent.
- If you have carpet, use a vacuum that has a special filter like a HEPA (High Efficiency Particulate Air) to trap those smaller particles from the carpet, and be sure to change it as needed per the manufacturer's instructions.
- If your allergies are severe enough, consider replacing all carpet with hardwood or other non-fabric floor coverings.
- All window coverings, whether fabric or other hard material, should be maintained as clean and dust-free as possible.

- If you don't have one, consider installing a venting system in your existing heating and air-conditioning system that filters the air coming in and out of your home.
- Be aware that furniture and other objects in your home, like books and magazines, can harbor dust, dust mites, and pet dander. Dust frequently or remove books and magazines. Replace furniture made with fabric covering with furniture made out of easier-to-clean materials, such as leather, vinyl, or wood. If you can not replace your furniture be sure to keep it clean. You can decide what to do with your precious kitty or 'Spot.'
- Nasal congestion for allergy sufferers is often due to local histamine production resulting in increased mucus production. Daily nasal saline rinses assist in ridding the nasal passages of offending allergens and clearing congestion.
- Finally, try to stem the tide of the worst bedroom offender—the dust mite allergen. If you have been sleeping on the same mattress for more than ten years, it just might be time to consider replacing it with a new one. Over a ten-year period, your mattress can swell to twice its weight with the insidious invasion of the dust mite.

The body's metabolism decreases at night; therefore your gastrointestinal tract cannot handle as efficiently a meal eaten late at night or just before bedtime. In addition, a large, heavy, spicy, fatty meal taxes your digestive system. The situation is worse in part for the GERD sufferer because in reflux disease, it has been shown that the lower esophageal sphincter (LES) is not as competent as in healthier individuals. The LES prevents the acidic contents of the stomach from regurgitating back up into the esophagus. Therefore, additional tips to help GERD sufferers include:

- Eat small frequent (four to five) meals per day.
- Avoid spicy, rich, and fatty meals before bedtime.
- Garlic, onions, chilis, peanuts, peppers, and curry contain volatile oils that can interfere with digestion; consume with caution in a late-evening meal.
- Avoid alcohol intake because it can precipitate an acid reflux episode.
- Limit the intake of acidic foods such as tomatoes and citrus fruits.
- If you are susceptible to acid reflux, watch out for mints and cinnamon in your diet.
- Get into the habit of avoiding mealtimes within four hours of your bedtime.
- Although they are almost universal favorite foods, limit the amount of chocolate and caffeine in your diet, especially in the few hours before bedtime. Coffee decreases pressure in the LES, contributing to reflux. For you hard-core regular coffee drinkers, perhaps try switching to a caffeine-free herbal coffee; start your weaning off caffeine by first preparing a mixed blend containing an herbal coffee with your regular coffee, and then over the next couple of weeks, continue to wean yourself off of the regular coffee by reducing the proportion of regular coffee in the blend.
- Don't wear tight-fitting clothes around your abdomen.
- Elevate the head of your bed to the position of your comfort at night; avoid sleeping flat on your back.
- Effectively manage your stress.
- Work with your primary care provider to establish a treatment plan that works for you.

Learn to rest in contentment. The apostle Paul in his letter to the Philippians encourages them not to let circumstance, good or bad, dictate their level of contentment in life. "For I have learned in whatever state I am, to be content: I know how to be abased, and I know how to abound. Everywhere and in all things I have learned both to be full and to be hungry, both to abound and to suffer need" (Phil. 4:11–12 NKJV).

Do not go to bed angry, and ask God's forgiveness for conscious and unconscious sin so that you can rest and sleep with a quiet peaceful conscience. The apostle Paul acknowledged that at times it is okay to be angry, but he admonishes:

> Be angry, and do not sin: do not let the sun go down on your wrath … (Eph. 4:26)

> And be kind to one another, tenderhearted, forgiving one another, even as God in Christ forgave you. (Eph. 4:32 NKJV)

Try to maintain a zest for life that God intended us all to have, including being optimistic about your future because you know who holds your future and you know who holds your hand.

"For I know the thoughts that I think toward you, says the LORD, thoughts of peace and not of evil, to give you a future and a hope" (Jer. 29:11 NKJV).

Exercising good sleep hygiene (engaging in healthy behaviors and practices that support a good night's sleep) is a part of displaying good spiritual discipline. This is both pleasing and honorable to God. Honoring the body refers to willfully raising up and respecting the sacred nature of the human body. This involves spiritual discipline. Good sleep habits or practices are specific actions that can be taken in order to honor and respect the body or temple of God as one prepares for sleep.

Spiritual discipline helps us to stay spiritually fit, able not only to put on the whole armor of God, but in addition helps us to develop patience and perseverance to run the race that is set before us.

Finally, pray before and after you sleep to thank and praise the one and only God of the universe for His wondrous medicinal gift of sleep; His provision, safety, and healing throughout the night; and His guidance and direction for the next day. Do you desire better sleep as a couple? Learn to pray not only as an individual but together as a couple. Couples who sincerely, openly, and routinely pray together are united together in one voice and one heart. A couple's prayer can be recited at bedtime when work and other commitments permit retiring to sleep at the same time, or you can choose one or more regular times during the day as your individual schedules permit. Before you start to pray, ask each other for prayer requests. As a practical matter, choose a position that is comfortable for both of you, either standing, kneeling, sitting, hugging, or lying in bed—holding hands or facing each other.

An Evening Prayer:

> Father, God in Heaven and Lord over all the earth …
> Thank You for watching over me and taking the best care of me and my loved ones today and every day.
> Thank You for the many ways You have shown Your lovingkindness to me all day long. Thank You, always, for Your divine provision and protection.
> I praise and magnify Your holy name for keeping me in Your love and care throughout this day. I pray that as I drift

off to sleep, put my heart and mind at ease. Let my mind reflect back, rejoice, and give thanks for all Your goodness to me.

Give me sweet and peaceful rest and restoration in order that I may awake restored and refreshed—fully recharged to serve You all the day through.

I praise You for the wonderful promise in Psalm 121:3–4: "He who keeps (me) ... will neither slumber nor sleep."

Amen

As you fall asleep, meditate on Deuteronomy 33:27: "The eternal God is your refuge, and underneath are His everlasting arms."

A Morning Prayer:

Father, God in Heaven and Lord over all the earth ...

Thank You for waking me up to a new morning with the privilege today of giving You all the glory in service to You! Let me begin this day with rejoicing, thanksgiving, and praise to You in my heart and on my lips for safely keeping me through another night.

Praise You for the promise in Your Word that Your lovingkindnesses never cease and Your compassions never fail, but are new every morning.

Help me to find new blessings every day and be thankful always for Your unconditional love and mercy.

Thank You for being ever watchful over me, even in the deepest part of the night. Help me to keep You uppermost in all my thoughts and every meditation of my heart. Help me to magnify and glorify Your great name in all that I do and say. I commit this day to You—in Jesus' wonderful name I pray.

Amen

In this chapter you were provided a long list of good sleep hygiene tips that work for most healthy normal adults. This list may seem a bit daunting to attempt all at once, but do not be overwhelmed; such an approach is not necessary. Good sleep habits are quite individual. Review the list and be realistic in choosing just a few tips that would be quick and easy for you to adopt right away in establishing good sleep hygiene. Your chosen subset of tips should be ones that you are willing to follow through with and use in your current living situation in order to make important and necessary lifestyle change. If there is a tip that you really know that you should adopt but you are struggling with carrying out the advice, seek help. You can proceed as time goes on adding those sleep habits to your diet and daily routine that will on most days help you obtain a good night's sleep.

Learning to properly take full advantage of God's many provisions involves the willingness to undergo personal change. For those who have problems regularly obtaining the best that proper sleep has to offer, they must often first embark on a journey to remove the cause of the insomnia by changing their lifestyle. For those suffering from chronic insomnia, adopting important lifestyle changes could be the initial key to obtaining the much-needed sleep that appears to be so elusive.

CHAPTER 9

Complementary and Alternative Therapies for a Good Night's Sleep

According to national survey data from the 2002 National Health Interview Survey (NHIS) conducted by the National Center for Health Statistics of the Centers for Disease Control and Prevention, over 17 percent of adults reported trouble sleeping or insomnia in the twelve months prior to the survey. Of those with insomnia or trouble sleeping, 4.5 percent—more than 1.6 million adults—used some form of complementary and alternative medicine/therapies (CAM or CAT) to treat their condition. Many people turn to CAT because conventional treatments have not worked for them, they lack confidence in conventional treatments, they prefer to go the "natural" route, or they understand and appreciate that there is still some lack of knowledge and uncertainty about the long-term effects of certain conventional treatments.

Although a list of CAT is provided below, a word of caution must be given. To date, comparison of these treatments, either with each other or with conventional therapies, has been difficult because many studies have not adequately defined insomnia, they contained a study sample that was too small, they lacked control groups, or there was no randomization of subjects into either treatment or control group. In addition, many CAT have yet to be tested on elderly subjects. As a result of these limitations in study design and generalizing the results of trials of these treatments, a definitive conclusion about the effectiveness of these therapies is difficult.

In addition, some interventions, such as aromatherapy and alternative sedatives, because of safety concerns may be contraindicated in specific patient populations such as the critically ill. Other therapies, such as progressive muscle relaxation and biofeedback, may be too difficult for these patients to perform. Massage, music therapy, and therapeutic touch are generally safe for critically ill patients and should be routinely applied only by critical-care nurses who have received training on how to administer these specialized interventions.

Complementary and alternative therapies (CAT) used to treat insomnia and induce sleep include supplements, light therapy, white noise, acupuncture, relaxation, meditation, and exercise. Listed alphabetically below are descriptions of the most commonly used CAT for sleep.

Supplement CAT

Calcium and Magnesium— Studies by Hughes, Richter, & Hamada et al indicate that calcium and magnesium supplementation may improve lower esophageal sphincter (LES) tone. This is good news for gastroesophageal reflux disease (commonly known as GERD) sufferers. In GERD the LES (the ring of muscle between the esophagus and the stomach) is not as competent as in healthier individuals. This sphincter prevents the acidic contents of the stomach from regurgitating back up into the esophagus.

German Chamomile has been used to discourage nightmares and as a relaxing fragrance to induce sleep when brewed as a tea. It is a commonly used herb for the treatment of insomnia. The FDA considers chamomile to be safe, and the plant extract has no known adverse effects.

Panax or Korean Red Ginseng (as a monopreparation in-low doses and for less than six months) has been used reportedly for insomnia caused by prolonged anxiety. It is important to note that there are several types of ginseng not all of which have the same or similar effects, mode of action, or drug-herb/herb-drug interactions. Therefore, it is best to consult with a knowledgeable integrative healthcare practitioner before taking any ginseng supplements.

Hops—Claims related to their ability to ease mood and anxiety are related to their long history of use as a sedative-hypnotic; given their estrogenic effects, they are contraindicated in people with estrogen-sensitive tumors. Comprehensive and extensive study is needed to validate efficacy and dosage and characterize the specific benefits of any of the components of hops.

Jasmine as a tea has been used reportedly for its soothing and calming effect.

Lavender, used as a potpourri, incense, or spray, is well-known for its aromatherapeutic sedative effects.

Lemon Balm has mild sedative properties and can ease gastrointestinal upset. Iberogast is a specific combination product containing lemon balm that reportedly improves symptoms of dyspepsia. It is not recommended for use longer than four months.

Melatonin is a hormone synthesized by the pineal gland, which is located in the center of the brain in humans. It is released by the pineal gland in response to the absence of light. Animals, as well as plants, also produce it. It plays a critical role in the regulation of the sleep-wake cycle and other circadian rhythms. Melatonin has been studied as a possible treatment of circadian-rhythm disorders. It can help re-entrain the sleep cycle in jet lag and decrease the sleep disturbances caused by jet lag. Adverse effects of melatonin are minimal, except in the case where an individual has epilepsy and is taking the anticoagulant warfarin. In addition, chronic melatonin use may have a mild skin-darkening effect in some susceptible individuals. Melatonin may not work for everyone. According to Wyatt et al. 2006, it was found that for healthy young adult subjects, melatonin was only effective during the times of day when the brain's internal clock was not already releasing its own supply of melatonin. Long-term studies are still needed to determine its true efficacy and toxicity. A study by Kandil, Mousa, El-Gendy, and Abbas, 2010 demonstrated that melatonin was useful as an adjunct treatment for gastro-esophageal reflux disease (commonly referred to as GERD).

Passionflower—Certain extracts of this herb have been used for their sedative effects, but use of or working around this herb should be closely monitored because of potential adverse reactions, such as hypersensitivity vasculitis or occupational asthma.

Skullcap (Chinese)—Theoretically, when used with alcohol or other drugs with sedating properties, this supplement can cause additive therapeutic and adverse effects.

St. John's Wort—Although mostly used for its antidepressant effects, this herb has also been used for insomnia (and many other ailments); yet for these indications, the clinical efficacy has not been well-supported in the research literature. In addition, there is a significant additive effect if it is used in conjunction with other prescription antidepressants. Therefore, you know the drill for this herb as with all others: always consult with your primary health-care provider before taking any herbal preparation.

Valerian—The effects of rhizomes and the root of valerian (Valeriana officinalis) on sleep have been studied in individuals with sleep disorders. The constituents of valerian are thought to act as central nervous system depressants. Some studies have suggested that valerian (especially as a tea) is beneficial in assisting with sleep induction and sleep maintenance. However, many of these studies had significant research design weaknesses, and no duplicate studies have been performed to confirm their initial findings.

Valerian should not be used for more than six weeks at a time because of the risk of liver toxicity or cardiac dysfunction. In addition, valerian can have serious drug-herb interactions when used with benzodiazepines, such as Xanax. Therefore, as of this date, additional better-designed research is needed before any accepted conclusions can be made about the safety and effectiveness of valerian for insomnia.

Other, Non-Supplement CAT

Acupuncture is used in traditional Chinese medicine for the treatment of insomnia. Recent preliminary clinical trials of acupuncture have indicated improvements in sleep quality for people with insomnia. However, additional research is needed before the effectiveness of acupuncture is proved conclusively for the relief of insomnia. When performed correctly and safely by an appropriately certified and trained acupuncturist, this technique is considered very safe.

Reflexology involves applying pressure with the top or side of the thumb or finger to reflex points on the sole or palm and sides and top of each foot or hand for up to three seconds before moving to the next position or digit. Skillful technique is used to relax and invigorate the body.

Aromatherapy's effectiveness in relaxation draws from the fact that the olfactory (smelling) neurons are directly connected to the brain. Thus, when activated, these neurons can stimulate the release of hormones or other substances that enhance or induce sleep onset. Therapy may be administered through inhalation using candles or steam, or when massaging or bathing.

Biofeedback has proven to be a very useful intervention for insomnia, since it can help an individual learn to relax. It is a noninvasive technique in which people use signals from their own bodies to improve their health and performance. A person is taught to adjust certain internal physiologic measures to a preferred outcome by using techniques such as guided imagery or progressive muscle relaxation.

Cognitive-Behavioral Therapies (CBT) involve time-limited goal-oriented focused psychotherapy. Clients change the way they think and behave because they learn how to think differently and act positively even if their situation does not change. These therapies can incorporate biofeedback, relaxation and breathing techniques, sleep restriction, stimulus control inputs (relearning to associate bed with sleeping), and establishing a sleep schedule. They also employ the use of homework assignments to practice what has been learned in a session. Studies have shown CBT to be beneficial in the treatment of intermittent and chronic insomnia.

Recently researchers have found that cognitive-behavioral therapy (CBT), which generally most often includes sleep restriction (limiting the number of hours spent in bed sleeping), stimulus control instructions (reeducating and relearning to associate bed with sleep), biofeedback, and relaxation techniques, in many cases improves sleep or problems with acute or chronic primary insomnia better than prescription medications.

Light Therapy (blue, red and violet) has proven useful in medicine as a treatment for seasonal affective disorder (SAD), a type of depression also known as "winter depression," resulting from a lack exposure to natural sunlight. In addition, twenty minutes of bright-light therapy has been used to reset one's biological clock when used for a few days immediately upon awakening. Caution: one should see an eye-care specialist to make sure that one does not have retinal disease before starting light therapy.

Massage, particularly therapeutic massage, can help with sleep disorders that have a neuromuscular origin, such as stress, pain, tension, or involuntary muscle contractions, such as restless legs syndrome. This method of massage relaxes the muscles and assists with improved blood flow. A therapeutic back massage reduces nerve irritation by enhancing production of pain-killing endorphins.

Common therapeutic massage techniques include:

Swedish massage—a smooth, flowing style that improves overall relaxation, circulation, and range of movement, and relieves muscular tension.

Deep-tissue or neuromuscular massage—a technique that penetrates down to the connective tissue layer, reaching tendons, ligaments, and nerves. Tension is released by massaging certain trigger points. This form of massage also breaks down adhesions and reduces inflammation which singly or together can cause pain.

Sports massage—involves the massage of specific muscles, tendons, and ligaments to improve athletic performance.

Infant massage has been shown to result in better sleep patterns and less crying in this age group. In addition, the calming touch of a parent during massage can provide a valuable opportunity to soothe and nurture one's baby. Some newborns may even develop a more regular sleep cycle.

Meditation or quieting the mind for twenty to thirty minutes can block or stop intrusive thoughts that contribute to problems with insomnia. Studies (Massion and Teas et al. 1995; Tooley, Armstrong, Norman, and Sali 2000; Harinath, Malhotra, Pal, Prasad, and Rai et al. 2004) have shown that regular meditation practice, either alone or in combination with the practice of yoga, results in higher blood levels of the sleep-regulating hormone melatonin.

Motion Therapies past studies (Harinath and Rai et al. 2004) have shown that tai chi and yoga can be used to improve sleep in older adults. It is well recognized that consistent regular exercise deepens sleep in young adults with or without sleep disorders. Recent studies show that even the low-to-moderate tai chi and yoga practices enhance sleep quality in older persons and cancer patients with sleep problems, respectively (Neuendorf, Wahbeh, Chamine, Yu, Hutchison and Oken, 2015).

Tai chi was originally a popular martial art from ancient China. It is now practiced throughout the world as an effective exercise for health. It teaches a series of fluid, gentle, and graceful circular movements, relaxed and slow in tempo. It also encompasses isometric exercise, specific breathing, relaxation, stretching, and correct body posture. When practicing tai chi, one focuses on the movements and the coordination of the body. The mental training in tai chi will enhance clarity of the mind, improve relaxation, and uplift mood.

Yoga in its various forms has three essential components: stretching exercise, breathing, and meditation. Regular practice of all three components results in a strong healthy body. For problems with sleep, the specific benefits of yoga include improvement in muscle relaxation; increased physical endurance, strength, and flexibility; mental stress reduction; and chronic pain management.

Music Therapy is known to have healing and relaxing effects. These effects appear to be mediated through neurotransmitters and neurohormones. It is used clinically to reduce stress, agitation, and anxiety and improve an individual's quality of life. Music therapy strategies include singing, drumming, listening to a quiet recording, and moving to music. A strategy using what is called "brain music," which matches music to an individual's specialized brain-wave patterns, reportedly improves sleep in people suffering from insomnia.

Relaxation Techniques, such as progressive muscle relaxation are aimed at relaxing the muscles. This is of therapeutic benefit because increased muscle tension can interfere with sleep and cause insomnia. Although most anyone can learn these techniques, it usually takes at least three weeks or more to sufficiently master them in order to help ease symptoms of insomnia.

Progressive muscle relaxation can relax muscle spasms and relieve muscle tension, thereby improving general muscle tone, relieving mental and physical fatigue, and promoting deep relaxation and stress reduction.

Visualization has been very helpful in getting individuals to relax. Performing this technique in the half hour before sleep can help make it easier for people to fall off to sleep.

White Noise masks or blocks other noises and sounds that may be disturbing to hear. It includes ocean or nature sounds, such as sea waves, gentle waterfalls, or sounds of the forest or other very soothing and quieting sounds or music.

Health problems associated with meditation and relaxation exercise are very rare. Yet relaxation exercises that involve abdominal tensing could cause problems for individuals with severe cardiovascular disease, or meditation could be problematic for individuals with psychosis or epilepsy. Certain yoga postures (poses) can put strain on the neck and result in non-intentional basilar (located at the base of the skull) or vertebral (located in the neck) artery occlusion.

When investigating the use of CAT, don't be fooled into believing that all these therapies are benign. Don't assume any therapy is safe just because it's labeled "natural," especially herbal or other dietary supplements. Beware of commercial claims of what herbal products can do. The current FDA guidelines allow for general health and wellness claims for these manufacturers. Any specific medical claims to treat, cure, or prevent specific medical conditions or disease must have prior evaluation and approval by the FDA. Look for scientific-based sources of information. Be leery of advertising that promises a cure-all or miracle cure, a medical breakthrough, or some other new medical discovery. When selecting a brand, choose one that lists the herb's common and scientific name, the name and address of the manufacturer, the batch and lot number, the expiration date, dosage guidelines, and potential side effects.

Before purchasing any supplement, you should consult with a nutritionist, herbalist, doctor, pharmacist, or certified integrative health-care specialist. Before deciding on a particular complementary or alternative therapy, you should learn as much as you can about that therapy. Start by asking certain questions, such as those that follow.

- What kind of track record does this form of therapy have in treating my condition?
- Is this treatment safe? What are the risks and benefits? What are the side effects?
- How many people with my sleep problem/disorder successfully use this form of therapy?
- How long has this therapy been successfully used for my particular condition?
- What does this therapy involve? What should I expect to happen when I use this therapy?
- What kind of facilities and providers will I be using with this therapy?
- Are the facilities clean, and is their equipment up-to-date and in proper working order?
- Are the providers experienced and properly trained, licensed, or certified? Are their diplomas or resumes available for review at their facility?

Always consult with your primary health-care provider before using any complementary and alternative therapeutic approach, even if you think he or she will disapprove or discourage you. As time goes on, conventional primary-care providers are becoming more open to learning about different treatments as complementary and alternative medicine (CAM) itself is becoming more popular. In addition, you want to avoid any serious negative interactions between CAM and any other conventional medicine that you are currently taking.

If you experience side effects such as shortness of breath, chest pain, rapid heartbeat, anxiety, nausea, vomiting, abdominal pain, diarrhea or skin rashes, or any other disturbing sign or symptom, barring any added rebound or other negative effect from abruptly discontinuing the herbal product, stop taking the herbal product and notify your primary-care provider immediately.

Foods that Promote Sleep

Sleep-promoting foods generally contain the essential amino acid tryptophan, which the body converts to serotonin, the neurotransmitter that slows down nerve traffic, which when converted to melatonin increases the deep-sleep stages and REM sleep. Tryptophan is called an essential amino acid because the body cannot manufacture it.

Foods high in the sleep-inducing amino acid tryptophan include:

- dairy products: cottage cheese, cheese, milk
- soy products: soy milk, tofu, soybean nuts
- seafood: tuna, halibut
- poultry: turkey
- whole grains: whole wheat, brown rice, buckwheat, oats (cereals such as oatmeal)
- beans, hummus, lentils
- hazelnuts, peanuts, walnuts, almonds
- egg whites

- dried fruit: figs, dates, berries, apricots
- fresh fruit: bananas
- leafy-green vegetables: lettuce*, bok choy
- sesame seeds, sunflower seeds
- spices: dill, sage, basil
- honey

*A special note about lettuce as a sleep-inducer. Ancient Egyptians used wild lettuce stem extract to induce sleep. Outside of the United States, it has been used for a long time to reportedly promote healthy sleep. This is because lettuce contains an opium-related substance, lactucarium, and traces of the antispasmotic agent hyoscyamine (the latter can have a side effect of drowsiness). Claims have been made that the two in combination help induce sleep.

Great sleep-inducing bedtime snacks are high in complex carbohydrates and calcium and medium to low in protein. These snacks should be eaten about one hour before bedtime because this is the time it takes for the tryptophan to reach the brain. Some examples include:

- apple pie and ice cream (my favorite)
- whole-grain cereal with milk
- hazelnuts and tofu
- oatmeal and raisin cookies, and a glass of milk
- peanut butter sandwich, ground sesame seeds

Remember: eat fresh, wake refreshed—eat light, sleep tight!

CHAPTER 10

A Hard Day's Night: How Do Shift Workers Manage?

Not everyone in our modern society can work the proverbial nine-to-five. In order to keep our society up and running, it is necessary to employ shift work. The primary reason that shift work is difficult for many people and can become a challenge to achieving and maintaining a healthy lifestyle is because our bodies are very sensitive to small changes in circadian rhythm. As a nation we sleep one hour less than we did fifty years ago and one and a half hours less than we did seventy-five years ago. Many of our institutions, such as hospitals, police, and fire must operate twenty-four hours a day, seven days a week. Today's health-care worker sleeps on the average only 6.8 hours on weeknights. This is one hour less than the allotment recommended as needed by the National Sleep Foundation. The health-care workplace plays a significant part in this blame.

There is strong evidence that shift work contributes to sleep disorders and that shift and night workers obtain less sleep than dayworkers. As with all the other sleep-deprived in our society, these workers are more likely to suffer from obesity, diabetes, cardiovascular, psychiatric, and gastrointestinal disease, and impaired immunity. Staying awake for a twenty-four-hour shift is equivalent to being legally drunk or having a 0.1 percent blood alcohol level.

One study of 79,000 nurses (from the Nurses' Health Study an ongoing prospective cohort of US female nurses first started in 1976) over a four-year period found after adjusting for risk factors such as smoking, BMI, hypertension, lipids, alcohol use, and physical activity, a modest dose-response relationship between coronary artery disease and shift work. Study findings indicated that 6 or more years of night shift work may increase the risk of CHD in women. Weight gain (the average was fifteen pounds) was more common in night-shift than day-shift nurses who were followed for five years. Later studies factoring in the putative effects of other cardiovascular risk factors such as psychosocial job strain, pyschobehavioral response to job strain or burnout, and social isolation resulted in similar findings (Kawachi, Graham, Colditz, Stampfer, and Willett et al. 1995; Knutsson and Bøggild 2000; Gu, Han, Laden, Pan, Caporaso, Stampfer, Kawachi, Rexrode, and Willett, et al. 2015).

Although it is well-known that sleep deprivation is a major safety risk factor for shift workers employed in life-or-death health professions, major industrial accidents such as the Exxon Valdez oil spill, the Three Mile Island and Chernobyl nuclear power plant accidents were in part attributable to errors made by fatigued night-shift workers.

According to the National Transportation Safety Board (NTSB) investigative reports, Exxon had been cutting back on staff in order to save money prior to the Valdez spill (NTIS Report Number PB90-916405 Washington, D.C. 1990). This cost-saving measure required the remaining employees to put in longer hours. The NTSB's final report revealed that the oil spill would have been avoided had not an exhausted third mate made some horrible mistakes due to sleep deprivation and sleep debt. The third mate had slept only six hours in the forty-eight hours just prior to the accident. On the day of the accident, the captain temporarily turned over command of the tanker to the third mate and left the bridge. Subsequently the sleep-deprived third mate did not perceive dangers pointed out to him by the lookouts, nor did he notice when he took over command that the autopilot was still on.

The activated autopilot interfered with maneuvering commands given by the third mate, who was trying to avoid ice floes in the channels leading into Prince William Sound. When he finally noticed that the autopilot was on, he turned it off and tried to redirect the huge tanker, but it was too late. Despite all subsequent maneuvers, the tanker still ran aground. Cleanup efforts topped the $2 billion mark, and $6 billion in punitive damages were awarded.

At 4:00 a.m. March 28, 1979, on Three Mile Island near Harrisburg, Pennsylvania, a nuclear accident came dangerously close to becoming a catastrophic nuclear disaster. Earlier that morning plant operators failed to recognize that even though the reactor had automatically turned itself off due to a malfunctioning automatic valve that had closed, shutting off the water supply to the reactor's cooling system, the entire system was experiencing a dangerous loss of coolant, and the reactor was overheating. Some of the zirconium-alloy fuel cladding failed, fuel itself partially melted, and cladding reacted with steam to produce hydrogen vapor bubbles, which then escaped into the reactor building.

Coolant was not restored to the reactor core until more than six hours after the accident. By that time enough hydrogen had accumulated in the building to pose the threat of a low-level explosion. The building had been designed to seal automatically in the event of a pressure rise, but no rise occurred, and four hours were allowed to elapse before the building was sealed, during which time radioactive gases escaped into the atmosphere.

Total nuclear meltdown and contamination were avoided because the containment vessel prevented any significant buildup of radioactive gases from escaping into the environment. The damaged reactor took the next ten years to decontaminate and be restored to complete functioning order. According to several agencies and commissions investigating the accident, fatigue in the wee hours of the morning contributed to repeated human failures to correctly interpret, respond to, manage and control the situation.

The worst nuclear accident in history happened in Chernobyl, Russia, on April 12, 1986. In the early-morning hours the day of the accident, engineers at the nuclear station decided for a never-quite-understood reason to keep one of the four reactors running even though they had shut down that reactor's regulatory and emergency safety systems and withdrawn most of the control rods from the nuclear reactor's core. The engineers claimed they were attempting to conduct an experiment, albeit ill-conceived.

The occurrence of fatigue-related accidents has spilled over into other fields as well, such as aviation and space aeronautics. The US space shuttle *Challenger* disaster on January 28, 1986, killed seven astronauts, one of whom was a friend of mine from my circa-1980 days of the young adult crowd at Trinity Baptist Church in Los Angeles, California. The case of overly fatigued, sleep-deprived National Aeronautics and Space Administration (NASA) Mission Control managers, who exercised poor judgment and decision making, was considered an indirect attributable cause to the accident (Space Shuttle Challenger Accident Report Vol. 2, Appendix G, 1986). These managers decided to proceed with the launch despite icy conditions (low temperatures), under which crucial O-ring seals (there were only two) had seriously failed earlier that same morning. During testing, the temperature of the rubber O-rings remained significantly lower than that of the surrounding air. Because the ambient temperature was within launch parameters, the launch sequence was allowed to proceed. These key managers had been on duty since the very early-morning hours with less than two hours of sleep the night before. It was later determined that the likely cause of the explosion was the failure of one of the Viton® O-ring seals.

Both shift work and jet lag are considered circadian-rhythm sleep disorders. In the airline industry, accidents have occurred because of the dual effects of sleep deprivation and jet lag. On June 1, 1999, after landing at the Adams Field Airport in Little Rock, Arkansas, American Airlines Flight 1420 was involved in a fatal runway accident. The McDonnell Douglas MD-82 overran the end of the runway, passed through a chain-link security fence, plunged down an embankment, and crashed into an approach-light support structure at the airfield. The airplane was destroyed by impact forces and a post-crash fire. Although at the time of the accident thunderstorms and heavy rain were reported in the area, the final NTSB report listed flight-crew decision making regarding operations in adverse weather and pilot fatigue among the contributing causes. The 145 passengers and crew aboard the flight suffered numerous nonfatal injuries; however, there were eleven fatalities, which included the airplane's captain and ten passengers.

Even though shift workers sleep, eat, and work at different times of the day, the principles of good sleep hygiene still apply.

Management strategies to decrease the incidence of sleep deprivation and its related negative effects on shift workers' health and productivity could include implementing work schedule adjustments such as:

- Maintain at least a twelve-hour hiatus between shifts.
- Avoid early shift starts (before 7:00 a.m.).
- If shift rotation is required, employ a forward or clockwise rotation of shifts (days to evenings to nights and then back to days). It is important to note that when rotating shifts, the least beneficial rotation is counterclockwise (nights to evenings, evenings to days, or days to nights) because it is more difficult to make a counterclockwise change in one's biological clock. Let me explain further: a counterclockwise shift rotation is similar to traveling west to east, demanding a higher degree of alertness at a time when one's biological clock-dependent alertness is at its lowest point. A worker who is trying to adjust to a counterclockwise rotation (for instance, days to nights) may initially incur a rapidly accumulating sleep debt, along with experiencing a low level of clock-dependent alertness. Leaving the night shift and driving home under these conditions could be a recipe for disaster.
- Keep simple, consistent, and predictable schedules.
- Avoid permanent night-shift work.
- Limit the number of long work shifts in a week.
- Limit an individual to no more than five to seven consecutive workday shifts during any given period of time.
- For those required to work every weekend, occasionally schedule them for some two-day nonworking weekends.

For many individuals their diet just before bedtime plays a significant role in whether or not they obtain a restful night's sleep. This may be particularly important for shift workers and those who are suffering from jet lag. These individuals should eat meals with a higher concentration of protein and carbohydrates, rather than fried or difficult-to-digest foods, and avoid going to bed immediately after consuming a large meal.

Circadian rhythms, homeostatic sleep regulators (sleep duration, quality and wake time), and sleep inertia effects are mechanisms that have significant impact on cognitive (learning and memory) physical, physiologic, and emotional functioning. Hopefully there will be future scientific investigation comprised of well-designed and powered studies that probe further into the significance of these mechanisms which in turn will lead to informed discussion and the establishment of public, private and government policy and programs to address acute and chronic sleep loss and deprivation in shift workers. A safe assumption for future study is that these mechanistic factors probably have a greater impact on shift workers. Therefore, a main focus of this future research should be investigation of these mechanistic effects impact the quality and safety of healthcare delivery and the health and well-being of heath care shift workers.

Likewise, these effects should also be studied in shift workers who provide public and military services (police, fire-fighting, transportation and aviation, and the Armed Forces). The ultimate goal is to devise and implement evidence-based and effective management strategies and interventions for sleep loss and fatigue in shift workers.

CHAPTER 11

———◉———

Sleep Throughout the Life Cycle

Sleep in the Newborn and Young Infancy

Babies have a very high need for sleep in the first few months of life. During these first few months, healthy newborn babies sleep an average of eighteen hours a day. For many parents adjusting life to a newborn baby's sleep pattern can be a daunting task. However, most parents with a great deal of confidence and a lot of stick-to-itiveness can more than satisfactorily accomplish this task.

For the first year of life, a baby will spend most of his or her time sleeping and eating. For many new parents, the biggest challenge is twofold: ensuring sufficient nighttime sleep for themselves and also being able to put the baby back to sleep when sleep becomes disrupted. It is also a good idea to check to see if the baby's diaper is wet when his or her sleep is disrupted. It is important to keep supplies close at hand to change the baby's diaper as quickly as you can and put the baby right back to sleep. Teaching the baby to self-soothe in the middle of the night and fall back asleep will be an invaluable skill when addressing disrupted sleep as the baby grows older.

It is very important for parents to learn and understand their babies' sleeping needs and patterns as soon as possible. A key factor in developing a sleep schedule is to put baby down for naps at certain times of the day. This will help baby to be more peaceful and fall asleep at a predictable time each night. It is also essential to recognize certain signs that your baby is becoming sleepy. Yawning, rubbing his or her eyes, a blank stare, and making jerky movements may be signals that your baby is getting sleepy. Be watchful, make sure to comfort your baby, and try to put the baby down as soon as you first recognize these signs. Doing so will help your baby to nod off peacefully and calmly to sleep.

In addition, when developing a sleeping schedule for a newborn baby, attention must be paid to the fact that sleeping and eating go hand in hand for the newborn. In fact, hunger often interrupts a baby's sleep. Newborns need to eat on the average at least every three to four hours. Therefore, in order to ease the stress on parents and baby, it is important to manage the baby's sleeping and eating schedules. Breast-feeding before a nap or bedtime may encourage the baby to relax. A meal before bedtime can extend the amount of time that a baby will sleep before becoming hungry again and needing to be fed. To help avoid colic, which can disrupt a baby's sleep, babies (less than twelve months old) should not be fed low-fat cow's, rice, almond, or soy milk.

Holding, cuddling, and bonding while baby is sleeping in your arms will promote emotional, physical, and mental growth, as well as the baby's brain development. Parental therapeutic touch can be enhanced by learning baby massage. Too much noise, attention, and excitement, especially by strangers, can cause a baby to become overstimulated. Babies may often cry and seek out the breast for comfort when they experience this type of sensory overload. It is okay to withdraw, breast-feed, and allow baby to settle down and become more relaxed.

Safe and Healthy Sleep Habits

A baby's crib and sleepwear should provide for safe and healthy sleeping. Do not place a newborn or infant baby to sleep on an adult bed or couch. Lay your newborn or young infant down in a crib or a bassinet for naps and nighttime sleep. Furthermore, to reduce the risk of Sudden Infant Death Syndrome or SIDS, do not place baby on his or her stomach to sleep (the prone position); instead, place baby on his or her back in a safety-approved crib (no drop-down sides) with a firm mattress covered with a tight-fitting sheet (flannel is okay). Never place toys, stuffed animals, pillows, or any other objects inside the crib where baby is sleeping or within a baby's reach.

Keep baby's face uncovered; keeping this in mind, do not lay baby on pillows or prompted up with wedges or other positioning devices, covers or blankets. In other words, do not use loose or rolled blankets, quilts, throws, or other soft bedding on top or underneath baby or in and around baby's crib. It is probably best if the use of quilts and blankets are avoided altogether. Keep the room temperature comfortable, avoiding air drafts flowing through the room where baby sleeps. Dress baby in light pajamas to prevent overheating in the warmer months of the year yet do not overdress or over bundle baby in the colder months.

Transitioning the Baby to Sleep

To create the mood and emotional feel for nighttime sleep, put baby down in a slightly warm bedroom-like location, with soft dim lighting with no more than quiet or low-level ambient noise in the surrounding area so that baby can drift comfortably and peacefully off to sleep. Some babies prefer gentle motion, such as rocking, and others enjoy soft music or both; still others may like being swaddled or cuddled close in an infant carrier or sling. Parents may want to experiment with a variety of techniques for transitioning baby to sleep and choose the one that best fits the space in time between feeding and sleeping. Mastering the best technique will make baby's nap and nighttime sleeping much easier.

When developing a sleep training schedule and routine, it is most often not a good idea to allow older siblings or pets into the room where the baby is sleeping. It is not unusual to find that the baby may become distracted and focus on these baby-sleep-routine trespassers instead of putting his or her head down and going to sleep. Not surprisingly, a baby's interest may become so heightened that he or she may actually initiate interaction with these trespassers on his or her own!

Softly and quietly singing or humming nursery rhymes is a tried–and-true technique; it has stood the test of time and still works beautifully! When softly sung or played, these melodic tunes are, as the saying goes, music to their ears.

In order to obtain sufficient sleep for you and your newborn, be realistic. Remember that sweet dreams for everyone takes time, effort, routine, and support. Be sure to contact your baby's pediatrician if you have any concerns or unsettling nervousness about your baby's sleep. I know some readers may feel they have no support; however, I encourage everyone to remember that God's love through prayer and the fact that He knows all and sees all guarantees that He will never leave or forsake us.

"So do not worry, saying, 'What shall we eat?' or 'What shall we drink?' or 'What shall we wear?' For the pagans run after all these things, and your heavenly Father knows that you need them" (Matt. 6:31–32).

"Be anxious for nothing, but in everything by prayer and supplication (petition), with thanksgiving, let your requests be made known to God ... And my God shall supply all your need according to His riches in glory by Christ Jesus" (Phil. 4:6, 19 NKJV).

Sleep In the Toddler Age

As the newborn baby rapidly grows and develops, new challenges arise. Infant and toddler sleep concerns include helping them to develop safe and healthy sleep habits. After one year of age, a special or favorite object, like a small stuffed animal, toy, or blanket, may help signal it's time to sleep.

A simple consistent bedtime routine is best for the toddler. It is okay to vary the routine sometimes, but not often (variety is only the spice of life as they get much older). Once again timing is everything. Make sure you stay very close (within ten minutes or so) of the time for nighty-night and lights-out.

During the day providing ample opportunity for a young toddler to exercise his or her mind and body is a great way not only to help with growth and development, but also to help ensure that when it is bedtime, he or she is ready to settle down and go to sleep. Activities such as hide-and-seek, tumbling, coloring, drawing, painting, playing with blocks, or building forts are fun for toddlers, parents, and older brothers and sisters who may want to join in the fun. However, complementing these activities with sweet snacks or drinks within a couple of hours of bedtime is a no-no.

When a toddler becomes very resistant to his or her bedtime routine (hopefully, mostly on rare occasions), it is wise not to get into the battle of wills between you and your toddler. More often than not, this battle will only escalate, leaving you and your toddler frustrated and worn out. If toddlers insist they are not sleepy, tell them that this is fine, but it is still bedtime. Give permission to quietly play a safe, short, simple game in bed or sing to themselves until they fall asleep.

Watching action videos or scary stories just before bedtime should obviously be avoided. This is especially important because toddlers sometimes at night may struggle with fear of the dark or separation anxiety. Instead, choose stories or videos that use an "and everyone lives happily ever after" plot ending that will make the toddler have the warm happy fuzzies as he or she drifts off to sleep.

If your toddler continues to have trouble falling asleep because of anxiety or fear, a good idea may be to leave on a soft night-light or use a transitional object (familiarly known as a lovey). A lovey is an object that a child can use to aid in obtaining his or her sense of safety and security, thereby easing his or her anxiety.

A Child's Morning Prayer

> Through the night thy angels kept me
> From above while I was sleeping.
> Now I'm awake; I am aware
> You've kept me in Your tender care.
>
> Although there is more that I could say,
> I just thank You, Lord, for this brand-new day!

A Child's Evening Prayer

Though this day has ended
I trust, Lord, all my hurts you've mended.

I thank you that every naughty thing I've done
You have forgiven me through your Son.

I'm in your eternal arms for safekeeping.

Bless me, Lord, now while I'm sleeping.

Sleep in School-Age Children

According to the NSF's 2004 Sleep in America poll – Children
and Sleep almost one in five preschoolers (19%) and school-
age children (18%) snore. A snoring sound can be produced
by blockages due to enlarged tonsils or adenoids. Snoring can
also be a sign of a severe sleep disorder such as sleep apnea. If
your child snores regularly or loudly, stops breathing, gasps for
breath, or has to work very hard to breathe while sleeping, he or
she may have sleep apnea. Children with sleep apnea can stop
breathing several times or more an hour. These disruptions
interfere with a child sleeping well through the night. The lack
of good sleep, or perhaps the lack of enough oxygen during sleep,
are suspected to increase the risk for daytime sleepiness and
hyperactivity, as well as daytime learning problems, which can
lead to poor school performance. Unlike adults, young children
who become sleep-deprived are typically more active during the
day, with problems of inattention and inappropriate behavior.

Odd sensations in a child's legs may keep him or her up at night.
These uncomfortable feelings in the legs may be a symptom
of restless legs syndrome (RLS). This movement disorder is

characterized by an uncontrollable urge to move when at rest or even while trying to fall asleep in an effort to relieve these feelings of discomfort. The 2004 Sleep in America poll revealed that children who reported having an uncomfortable feeling in their legs slept an hour less at least a few times a week and were twice as likely to wake up during the night as children without these complaints. A significant percentage of children commonly reported waking during the night and complained of sleep problems (Mindell, Meltzer, Carskadon, and Chervin, 2009). The precise cause of restless legs syndrome is unknown. It can be related to iron deficiency or associated with kidney or certain neurological diseases. Familial occurrence is thought to have a genetic link or component attached to its incidence. As with any sleep disorder, RLS in children should be referred to a pediatrician or a sleep specialist.

In addition to the distractions of television, video games, cell phone use, older siblings, and the need to rebel against bedtime, sleep itself can be a problem for many children. Sleep problems in children can range from trouble falling asleep to night terrors.

Sleep-Smart Tips for School-Age Children and Their Parents

- Set regularly scheduled bedtimes. Children and teens don't get enough sleep. According to the NSF 2006 Poll 60 percent of children under the age of eighteen complained of feeling tired during the day, and 15 percent reported falling asleep at school during the day. As parents we need to set regular bedtimes, even for teens, to help them get enough rest.
- Exercise. Physical activity eases tension and helps children and teens relax. If a child does not play a sport, then playing outside after school or taking a long walk

with a parent after dinner can help him or her manage stress.

- Eat regularly scheduled healthy meals. Scheduling and maintaining regular, healthy meal plans helps children to cope with stress. Mealtimes are even better when the whole family sits down to eat together. In addition, keep children away from caffeine in the hours before bedtime.

- Engage your children in meaningful conversation. Communicate with your child often and ask him or her how things are going. If your child seems stressed or talks about feeling like he or she has too much to do, ask how you can help. Brainstorm ways that you can solve problems together. For example, if your child feels he or she has a big problem, talk about how you might be able to break it up into smaller pieces and solve them one at a time.

- Limit activities. Choose one or two activities that your child enjoys, and explore other interests at a more appropriate opportune time. You will not jeopardize raising a well-rounded child if you don't place him or her at the same time in soccer, piano, dance, art classes, and other worthwhile activities. Overloading your child with too many activities might be more than your child can handle.

- Establish and maintain regular routines and rituals. Research and reviews by Barbara Fiese, PhD, of Syracuse University published in 2002 and 2006 demonstrated that organized, regular routines and rituals create a sense of safety and security for children, help organize family life, and enhance the well-being of families, particularly the children. Furthermore, in families with set routines the children slept better, were healthier overall, performed better in school and suffered from fewer respiratory illnesses.

- Pray for each other in the morning and in the evening—
  and pray out loud, acknowledging and professing your
  love and support for one another. Pray that through
  God's Holy Spirit, you are both united as one.

  "Can two walk together unless they be agreed?" (Amos 3:3
  NKJV).

- Pray for the two of you to have a servant's heart. God
  wants us to serve others, not to be served. Jesus stated
  in the Gospel of Mark 10:14, "Even the Son of Man did
  not come to be served, but to serve."
- Pray for God's protection over you and your household,
  extended family, and others. Pray for God's guidance, not
  only for you as a couple, your family, and extended family,
  but also for your governmental leaders. There is a saying
  that goes like this: "A couple that prays together stays
  together." Prayer is a couple's opportunity to connect
  together through the power of the Holy Spirit with God,
  our Father and Creator. It is a wonderful blessing and
  privilege to be able to approach Him together. Praying
  together will encourage you to grow spiritually together
  as one.

Sleep in Adolescence

Sleep-deprived parents may have become so accustomed to
their own chronic fatigue that they may not recognize sleep
problems in their school-age children and teens. Another myth
that many parents and teens hold is that it is often necessary
that teens must stay up late to study to be successful in school.
Yet according to the National Sleep Foundation's (NSF) 2006
Sleep in America poll, students who got optimum sleep (9 +
hours) reported performing better in school, with 34 percent

A grades and 46 percent reporting B to A grades versus 18 percent who reported insufficient (less than 8 hours) amount of sleep. This result supports other studies that show A and B students report going to bed earlier and getting more sleep than students with poorer grades.

Epidemiological research on "normal" sleep patterns and amounts demonstrate that adolescents average only seven to seven and a half hours of sleep per night. However, research on sleep-wakefulness patterns reveals that adolescent sleep needs do not decline significantly and that optimal sleep amounts remain about nine hours into late adolescence.

Does burning the midnight oil really help students succeed more in school? More than 50 percent of fatal traffic accidents involve teen-age drivers. How much has sleep deprivation in the teenage years contributed to this statistic? Most adolescents need at least eight and a half hours of sleep each night, according to the NSF's 2006 Sleep in America poll. The poll reports that only 15 percent of young people get this amount of sleep, with 25 percent of teens getting less than seven hours. Currently in the state of Arizona, it is illegal to drive while sleep-deprived.

Sleep disorders that emerge and become especially prevalent in adolescence are delayed-sleep phase syndrome and narcolepsy.

Advice for Sleep-Smart Parents of Adolescent Teens

Parents must realize that signs of sleep deprivation commonly appear in the morning, rather than at night. They must dispel the misconception that it is "normal" to be sleepy for the first hour after waking up or that their teen is just bored or apathetic about school, causing him or her to fall asleep in class, arrive late to school, or underperform. A significant number of teens find it difficult to fall asleep before 11:00 p.m. and then rise and shine (and give God the glory) by 8:00 a.m. the next morning—a sleep pattern that is worse in males than in females. In fact, these signs, along with others such as irritability and dependency on caffeine, indicate that teens might be suffering from sleep deprivation, and their parents should not be mistaken by the burst of energy they get in the evening.

It is this flip-flop behavior of teens that often fools parents into believing that their children are well-rested. Therefore, parents should look for signs of daytime sleepiness, especially in the morning, by paying attention to teen caffeine consumption, napping, and mood. Because the circadian sleep rhythms of adolescents compel them to go to bed later and arise later, parents might mistakenly view their teens' obstinacy about adhering to school days' bedtime as just normal teenage behavior, rather than as an aspect of their biology.

Parents and teens both should know what good sleep entails and take advantage of the benefits of making and adhering to a plan that promotes good sleep. This way both will do a better job making choices about what are truly essential activities in which to be involved. Help your teen to establish consistent sleep and wake schedules. Set a good example: get enough sleep and talk to your teen about the importance of sleep. Finally, remove sleep detractors from the bedroom—put the TV and computer in a common room instead of the teen's bedroom, or at least make a pact that these devices are turned off at a specific time.

Along with preparing teens for life's challenges as they grow and mature, successful stress management can help teens get their necessary sleep at night. Prioritize. Prioritize. Plan. Each year sit down and discuss what's most important in your teen's life, whether it is school, grades, sports, friends, a job, or some other venture. Then, during times of stress, use your list of priorities to decide what can be eliminated or put on hold for a while. For example, if playing on the high school football team is more important to your teen than his part-time job, he might want to talk to his boss about not working during football season. Set limits. Before your teen takes a job, the work schedule and the number of work hours needs to be negotiated, based on homework, other activities, financial need, and last but not least, your individual teen's biological makeup.

In addition, the community at large (especially school-board curriculum planners, sports instructors, and driver-education instructors) is responsible for ensuring that school start times, homework load, and extracurricular activity schedules affecting school-age children and older teens' lives are developed and set in a healthy and realistic way. Decisions made on these issues should be informed by sleep anatomy and physiology, a balanced perspective on teen developmental needs, and teens' social and behavioral concerns.

Here are some easy steps for teens to help improve their quantity and quality of sleep.

- Strive to get at least eight hours of sleep each night.
- Go to bed at the same time each night, and get up at the same time each morning.
- Prepare for the next school day the night before by making lunch, laying out your clothes, showering, and packing up your schoolwork. This will allow you to set a later morning awake time and still not prevent you from getting to your first morning class on time.
- Eat more healthily, avoiding frequent intake of foods such as caffeinated sodas and chocolate.

- Find time to relax and unwind after a busy school day and before you go to bed; turn off the cell phone and the television, put down the electronic game controls, and eliminate all other technology distractions.
- Avoid any late evening/early night (after 9:00 p.m.) sports participation.
- Avoid all-nighters by planning sufficient study necessary to prepare for exams and research efforts to complete school projects on time.
- If you have trouble falling asleep, keep a writing pad near your bedside as a place to jot down all the things that are running through your mind.
- Turn your bedroom into a soothing and relaxing place for sleep.
- Avoid caffeine altogether. Under no circumstances abuse drugs or alcohol.
- Turn on all the lights and open all the shades once you wake up in the morning.
- Choose more healthy eating choices when you must eat away from home.
- If you continue to have sleeping problems, keep a sleep log for yourself.

Symptoms of sleep deprivation in teens can include:

- daytime yawning
- dozing off in morning classes or being sleepier than one would like to be
- having trouble getting out of bed in the morning
- taking more than twenty minutes to fall asleep at night
- falling asleep while participating in favored activities or those you want to do
- missing preferred or interesting activities because of feeling too tired or sleepy

- falling asleep while driving
- needing to drink coffee to stay awake
- frequent headaches
- feeling irritable or moody or on edge all or most of the time
- feeling too tired to socialize with friends
- clumsiness
- having difficulty focusing, concentrating, or just thinking clearly
- having thoughts that at times appear to wander or be disconnected
- having to sleep in late on the weekends
- having seven o'clock in the morning feel like the middle of the night

The National Institutes of Health (NIH) provides a free supplementary curriculum on sleep development for ninth-through twelfth-grade biology students. The curriculum, entitled "Sleep, Sleep Disorders, and Biological Rhythms," is available for science teachers and school administrators upon request in print form, as well as online at: http://www.science. education.nih.gov/customers.nsf/highschool.htm or http://www. science.education.nih.gov/supplements/nih3/sleep/default.htm.

Advice for Sleep-Smart Adolescent Teens

Besides the toddler and young child age, the teenage years define one of the most active physical and emotional periods of growth in life. As the next stage of life - young adulthood approaches opportunities to be involved in various activities can come fast and furious as also will the highs and lows, joys, and pressures that they bring.

For most teenagers getting enough food and exercise is no problem at all. However, faced with the demands of early school start times, homework, clubs, sports, after-school activities (including work for some teens), and of course, dating – getting adequate amounts of sleep on school nights can be a real challenge. Savvy teens, already know this, however, for others the question becomes: What can I do about being so sleep deprived and feeling that I have to catch up on missed sleep on the weekends?

Before providing some good suggestions that can help teens meet important sleep needs for their growing bodies, keep themselves up beat and their minds at ease, here are a few facts:

Sleep is essential to everyone's health and well-being, as important as the air we breathe, the water we drink, and the food we eat. Proper sleep helps us all to manage stress, especially the stress of being a teenager or the parent(s) of a teenager. Sleepiness can make it difficult to get along with family and friends and interfere with one's academic performance and sports performance on the court, track or field.

Generally-speaking during adolescence circadian sleep patterns for sleep and wakefulness shift toward later times. This means it comes natural for many adolescents not to be able to fall asleep before 11:00 p.m. and feel groggy (or even sad or cranky) if awakened prior to 8:00 a.m.

Sleep-deprived teens can become sad and/or apathetic which can lessen their ability and willingness to concentrate on important tasks such as schoolwork or car-driving. Moreover, persistent sleep-deprivation can limit your ability to listen, pay attention, concentrate and solve problems. As a consequence, not getting enough sleep, teens (as would any sleep-deprived person would) are more likely to have an accident, suffer injury or illness. Remember: A brain that is hungry for sleep will demand it and get it, even when you don't expect it.

Now the following are some suggestions:

Get adequate sleep by keeping a regular sleep-wake schedule on weekdays as well as on weekends, not varying you schedule by more than 1 hour. Establish a bedtime and wake-time routine and keep it. A consistent sleep schedule will help you feel less tired and will allow your body to get in sync and keep in sync with its natural sleep-wake patterns. Falling asleep at bedtime will be easier when keeping this type of routine.

Taking a mid-day nap may be next to impossible with your schedule but somehow try to fit in 15-20 minutes of down time or rest in order to get yourself through the rest of the day.

Engaging in regular exercise and physical activity will lead not only lead to better overall fitness but better quality sleep. Try as much as possible to avoid any strenuous exercise within 2-3 hours of your regular bed time.

The jury is still out and there is no consensus on the pros and cons of caffeine consumption; however, caffeine can disrupt sleep, therefore the consumption of caffeine-containing products such as coffee, black and green tea (including iced tea), energy drinks and bars, and chocolate (yes, chocolate) should be avoided in the evening.

No big lecture here about being an under-age substance user, just suffice it to say: don't smoke cigarettes, cigars or use any other nicotine-containing products and don't drink alcohol.

Don't go to bed hungry. It is best to avoid eating a heavy meal or snacks within 2 hours of your bedtime as this may interfere with sleeping soundly at night – and don't skip breakfast. A healthy high protein breakfast can sustain you throughout the rest of the day's activities and prevent you from having blood sugar swings which in a crunch may tempt you to eat or crave unhealthy snacks in order to get by until your next real meal. Do not eat a heavy meal, drink more than four ounces of fluid or exercise within 3-4 hours of your regular bedtime.

Include daily "wind down" time. Set aside up to 1 hour of quiet time before bedtime every night. He or she should use this time for calm and enjoyable activities, such as listening to quiet music, reading a book, or functions that let the mind and body relax. Television, computer games, any screen time (mobile devices), exercise, or heavy studying should not be part of quiet time. The last several minutes of quiet time activity may take place in the room where you sleep. The bed however, should be used only for sleeping insuring that a firm association of your bed with sleep will be built up in your head and become a part of your regular frame of mind.

Turn your bedroom into an inviting, clean, uncluttered, and relaxing environment conducive to sleep. Keep it quiet and a comfortable temperature (less than 75° F). Although, it may be tempting because your bed feels so comfortable and you feel so relaxed there, however, once again only use your bed for sleep not a place for reading, studying or playing. Try to avoid the television, computer (or other electronic devices) and the telephone in the hour before you go to bed. In particular this means do not leave your homework until the last minute before your bedtime.

Sleep During the College Years

Sleep disorders and insufficient sleep have a tremendous impact on school performance, health, and psychosocial development during the second decade of life. Living in residence halls with many other people or living off campus can make it difficult to get enough sleep. Other concerns, such as social life, academic life, and work can also inhibit good sleep patterns in college. The entire buzz atmosphere of college life lends itself to sleep problems.

Lack of sleep in college-age students can result in lack of concentration and growing inability to focus, with students finding themselves reading the same page over and over as their mind wanders. The tendency for risk-taking behavior also increases during this period of life. Interest in extreme sports is highest in the college-age population. The stress and strain of the demands of college can lower their immunity. Add this to close living arrangements, and the two together can place individuals in this age group at risk for many community-acquired respiratory illnesses. College-age students with chronic sleep deprivation are at a greater risk for depression and anxiety.

Educational Sleep Tips for College-Age Young Adults

- Sleep is energy-producing for the brain; therefore make sure you get enough of it and get it when you need it. Even mild daytime sleepiness can hurt your performance—on school exams as well as playing sports or video games. Lack of sleep can make you look and feel tired and depressed and make you respond irritably and angrily.
- Establish a regular bedtime- and waking-time schedule and resist the temptation to sleep in. Maintain this regular routine on the weekends and even on vacations. Don't frequently stray from your schedule, and never do so for two or more consecutive nights. If you must go off schedule, avoid delaying your bedtime by more than one hour, awaken the next day within two hours of your

regular schedule, and if you are sleepy during the day, take a short early-afternoon nap.

- Learn how much sleep you need to function at your best. You should awaken refreshed, not tired. Most adolescents need between eight and a half and nine and a half hours of sleep each night. Know when you need to get up in the morning, then calculate when you need to go to sleep to get at least eight and a half hours of sleep a night.
- Expose yourself to bright light as soon as possible in the morning, but avoid it in the evening. The light helps to signal to the brain when it should wake up and when it should prepare to sleep.
- Understand your circadian rhythm. Then you can try to maximize your schedule throughout the day according to your internal clock. For example, to compensate for your slump (sleepy) times throughout the day according to your internal clock, participate in stimulating activities or classes that are interactive, and avoid lecture classes or potentially unsafe activities, including driving.
- In the afternoon, stay away from coffee, colas with caffeine, and nicotine, which are all stimulants. Also avoid alcohol, which disrupts sleep. *Under no circumstances abuse drugs—this means recreational drug use is explicitly verboten!*
- Relax before going to bed. Avoid heavy reading, studying, and computer games within one hour of going to bed. Don't fall asleep in front of the television because flickering light and stimulating content can inhibit restful sleep. If you must work during the week, try to avoid working night hours. Even if you work late-evening hours, you will still need to plan time to relax and unwind before going to sleep.
- Don't pull all-nighters. Staying up late can greatly disrupt your sleep patterns and your ability to be alert

the next day and sometimes for the next few days. Getting the proper amount of sleep is the best thing you can do the few nights before a big test. All-nighters or late-night study sessions may give you more exam-cram time, but your ability to retain and recall will more than likely be negatively affected.

- Don't overlook the influence of college pressure and stress in your busy life. Balancing heavy academic loads with special activities, such as sports or externships, work, and having any semblance of a social life is nearly impossible to accomplish stress-free. The American College Health Association-National College Health Assessment continues to demonstrate stress as the #1 impediment to academic performance. Now may be the time to take advantage of using a daily planner or start to use the electronic calendar located on your cell phone or other mobile device to help keep you organized.

- Don't be ashamed or embarrassed to take advantage of support groups located on campus or in the community either. If you are having roommate concerns, try to work it out among yourselves as soon as possible. If this tactic does not work to your satisfaction, then get an impartial third party to mediate (e.g., residence assistants). Finally, nurturing yourself spiritually is an excellent way to help reduce your stress. Attend church regularly, pray, and get involved in a Bible-study fellowship that has college-age attendees like you. Don't allow being away from home for the first time or failure to fit in with this group or that one make you feel lonely. There is always something you can do to avoid this happening to you. Relax, pray, and ask God to guide you toward other individuals with whom you can relate well and socialize, form study groups, and support one another. It may take some time and effort, but you can do it.

Sleep in Adult Women – A Look at Pregnancy and Menopause

Women from adolescence to postmenopause are underrepresented in studies on sleep and sleep disorders. Although sleep complaints are twice as prevalent in women, 75 percent of sleep research has been conducted in men. More sleep studies in the past five years have included women, but study limitations such as small sample sizes have not permitted valid and meaningful sex comparisons.

Understanding and providing appropriate sleep advice across the life cycle of the woman is important because the development of chronic insomnia has been linked to precipitating events. Both sleep apnea and restless legs syndrome have been shown to increase during pregnancy and menopause, but certain treatment options may be contraindicated or are not specific for women. It is important that advice and treatment options address the specific physical discomfort and interfering life events experienced by women.

Sleep in Childbearing-Age Women

During this time period, many women experience premenstrual daytime sleepiness, which is relieved once menses starts. This is probably due to sensitivity to the sedating effects of progesterone because the level of progesterone during this time is low. A rise in estrogen during the follicular phase of the menstrual cycle can cause an increase in REM sleep.

During the early luteal phase, progesterone begins to rise and acts to increase body temperature and blunt the circadian rhythm. Consequently, women tend to get sleepy earlier and wake up earlier because their melatonin rhythm is blunted.

All these sleep-related effects of hormonal changes during a woman's monthly cycle are often worse for women who suffer from premenstrual syndrome. Abdominal bloating is the number-one PMS complaint and a major contributor besides cramping to decreased nighttime sleep.

Sleep Tips for Childbearing-Age Women

- Get your proper amount of daily exercise, which we all should know by now promotes good health and sound sleep.
- Watch your daily salt intake. Steer clear of a high intake of processed foods and commercial seasoning preparations, of which the vast majority contain high amounts of sodium.
- Maintain adequate water intake to handle excess salt hidden in foods. Excess dietary sodium can lead to water retention.
- Watch your alcohol intake. Women metabolize alcohol differently from men, and during the premenstrual time frame, women may also be more sensitive to its effects.
- Watch your intake of refined sugar and sweets. Sugar is metabolized very quickly. Too much sugar, especially when not in conjunction with a well-balanced dinner or snack, can lead to a precipitous drop in blood sugar, which can wake you up at night.
- Take extra daily calcium. Many premenstrual symptoms resemble the symptoms of calcium deficiency. Calcium supplementation in doses as high as 1,200 mg per day have been shown by the third month of supplementation to decrease PMS symptoms. Calcium has a very modest sedating effect; therefore for sleep promotion, it perhaps should be taken at night. Excess calcium can cause kidney stones and other health problems; therefore check

with your primary care provider before deciding on the appropriate dose to take. Calcium should be taken with food to ensure proper absorption.

- Besides being a healthy evening snack, bananas tout a mild soporific effect through their stimulation of melatonin and serotonin production.
- For breast tenderness try taking chaste tree berry (Vitex) or applying cold packs to the breasts. Chaste tree berry has anti-inflammatory and progesterone-like properties, which may help relieve symptoms of PMS. A word of caution: current research data is scant on the long-term safety and clinical efficacy for the use of chasteberry in PMS symptom relief.
- Evening primrose oil, with its anti-inflammatory properties, has been reported to ease the symptoms of PMS.
- Ginger or juniper berry tea reportedly provide relief from menstrual cramps.
- A concoction of almond oil and chamomile rubbed on the abdomen reportedly eases menstrual cramps in some women.
- Finally, Grandma's and even perhaps your mom's old standby remedy of moist heat applied to the abdomen can do the trick to ease symptoms of PMS in many women (but be careful not to apply heat directly to the skin for too long).

Sleep During Pregnancy

For some mothers-to-be, especially first-time moms, sleep becomes a challenge in the first trimester. Adjusting to the mental and physical effects of the first trimester can be a challenge for some. Many first-time mothers may feel less energetic and should therefore schedule themselves for additional sleep. This extra sleep can help make pregnancy a more positive experience.

It is not uncommon for pregnant women to contend with sleep disturbances caused by nausea, back pain, and constantly getting up and running to the bathroom. The enlarging uterus can cause a cramped pelvic space for the bladder, leading to increased urgency that may require the pregnant woman to get up several times during the night to empty her bladder. These problems are mainly due to anxiety, stress, hormonal fluctuations, and physical discomfort. Some women develop restless legs syndrome (RLS), snoring, wild dreams, and insomnia (Manconi, Govoni, De Vito, Economou, Cesnik, Mollica, and Granieri 2004). As pregnancy progresses it may become difficult to find a comfortable sleeping position.

Trimester Effects on Sleep

Morning sickness is quite common in the first trimester of pregnancy. This may cause earlier-than-desired awakening in some women due to nausea. If this situation worsens, it can lead to a condition called hyperemesis gravidum.

Lack of energy and feeling sleepy or fatigued may be due to the soporific (sleep-inducing) and thermogenic (heat-producing) effects of high progesterone secretion from the placenta that occur during the first trimester.

As the body changes, discomfort can make it harder to fall and stay asleep. Breast tenderness can make the pregnant mother uncomfortable and make it difficult for stomach sleepers. As pregnancy progresses and the uterus enlarges, the diaphragm becomes restricted and breathing becomes more shallow; the intestines and esophageal sphincter are displaced upward, potentially causing esophageal reflux and complaints of heartburn, particularly in the supine position.

The second trimester usually provides some relief for the pregnant mom as hormones level off and most often nausea subsides. Nighttime trips to the bathroom are not as frequent because the enlarging uterus moves up from the pelvis into the abdomen, thus relieving bladder compression by the uterus.

The third trimester is the most sleep-challenged stage of pregnancy. Back aches and pain are associated with softening of the uterine ligaments and pelvic-hip joints loosening in preparation for birth. With back pain, muscle aches, fetal movement, the frequency of urination, inability to get comfortable, and exhaustion from trying to keep up with the demands of their normal schedules, some women find themselves struggling to stay awake. The weight of the baby also affects posture and can leave many women uncomfortable sleeping, walking, or sitting.

Many pregnant women begin snoring because of nasal congestion that blocks airways and increases in abdominal girth and the uterus that press on the diaphragm. If the blockage is severe, sleep apnea may result, characterized by loud snoring and periods of stopped breathing during sleep. Snoring can also lead to high blood pressure, which can put both the mother and fetus at risk.

A number of pregnant women develop restless legs syndrome during the third trimester. In fact, studies have linked restless legs syndrome to pre-pregnancy iron and/or folic acid deficiency (Lee, Zaffke & Barette-Beebe, 2001; Djokanovic, 2008). Fortunately, for most women restless legs syndrome goes away with childbirth.

Painful lower leg muscle cramps are fairly common both in the second and third trimester. These spasms occur most often at night and thus can disrupt sleep. Leg cramps are believed to be caused by an excess of phosphorus and a shortage of calcium circulating in the blood system.

More Pregnancy Sleep Tips

- Reduce stress and anxiety. Stress and anxiety are key culprits in preventing a good night's sleep. If necessary seek out a friend or a professional who can listen and help if there are issues in your life that are causing you to worry or feel upset. During this time it is very important to get the rest you need for your and your baby's optimum health.
- Drink plenty of fluids during the day, but cut down before bedtime to minimize frequent nighttime urination. Doing pelvic tilts called Kegel exercises before lying down can help decrease the number of bathroom breaks at night.
- If you need a light when heading off to the bathroom at night, use a night-light instead of overhead or bedside lighting. Use of a night-light will be less rousing and help you return to sleep quicker.
- Exercise regularly, which besides being essential for optimum health in general, during pregnancy will help you sleep, help with energy levels, and improve circulation (thus reducing nighttime leg cramps). Avoid exercising late in the day; exercise releases adrenaline into your body that can keep you awake at night.
- If leg cramps wake you up at night, try stretching prior to going to bed. Before going to bed, perform five to ten repetitions of alternately straightening the leg and then flexing the foot upwards. This can help prevent future lower leg cramping.

- Establish a consistent, soothing, and comforting evening routine. This will help you to relax and fall off to sleep with more ease. As bedtime approaches try a few soothing rituals. Drink a cup of caffeine-free tea or warm milk, read a chapter or two in a light not-too-overstimulating book, take a warm shower with a shower gel that has a gentle relaxing fragrance such as lavender or lemon-sage, get a shoulder massage, or practice your grandmother's hair-pampering tip: one hundred hairbrush strokes.

- Lie in the left-lateral supine position for rest and sleep. During the first trimester, start training yourself to sleep on the left side to improve blood flow and nutrients to the fetus and uterus. This will also optimize blood flow to the kidneys to get rid of waste and help with excess fluid retention. Avoid lying flat on your back for a long period of time.

- Watch carefully what you eat during pregnancy; maintain a well-balanced diet. Completely eliminate caffeine and alcohol to help prevent insomnia. If nausea is a problem, try eating frequent bland snacks (like crackers) throughout the day. Avoid meals close to bedtime, particularly if heartburn is a problem. Keep your stomach slightly full, which can help prevent nausea. Not only is this crucial for your and your baby's health, but getting the necessary nutrients will help keep you feeling satisfied and less prone to major nighttime snack attacks that may contribute to restlessness and insomnia when you go to sleep.

- After a meal do not recline for another one to two hours in order to prevent heartburn. If heartburn is a problem, sleep with your head elevated on pillows. Avoid spicy or acidic foods such as tomato products, citrus fruits or drinks, and fried foods, as they may worsen symptoms.

In addition, eat frequent (four to five) small meals throughout the day.

- Pregnancy is a time of additional energy demands; therefore it is a good idea to nap during the day. Although it can be difficult with other children around, take a short half-hour nap to help reduce fatigue, especially if you are not getting enough rest at night. Feel free to nap on the couch while an older child or children play quietly nearby. Finally, do not feel guilty if you need to sleep in or head off to bed early from time to time.

- Support your body with pillows! Use them wherever you may need them: between your knees for aching hips, under your belly for support, behind your back, underneath your legs and ankles, or under your head. For comfort try sleeping on your side with one pillow under your knee and another under your belly. You can use a special pregnancy body pillow or a regular pillow to support your body or to aid in comfort measures.

- If you wake up in the middle of the night or have trouble falling asleep, don't just lie there. Get up for a bit and read or do something not too stimulating. If insomnia persists schedule a visit with your health-care provider for advice and help. Hopefully during your visit you can learn about support groups to help with stress management and other concerns during pregnancy.

Sleep During the Postpartum Period

Much of the information we have on sleep during the postpartum period comes from the National Institutes of Health (NIH) National Center on Sleep Disorders research. A compilation of findings derived from sleep diaries indicate there is considerable sleep disturbance in the early postpartum period.

Sleep efficiency improves during the first year postpartum, but it is unclear because the information is gathered from self-reports whether sleep quantity and quality return to pre-pregnancy levels.

During the first three to four months postpartum, there is a relationship between sleep and mood. Increased disturbances in self-reported sleep, including decreased total sleep time, are associated with depressed mood postpartum.

Although most infants achieve sleep maturity by the second half of their first year, many still wake up during the night. Reasons for this include painful or uncomfortable stimuli provided by frequent nasal congestion, colds, or teething pain. In addition, reaching major developmental milestones, such as sitting, crawling, and walking, drive infants to practice their new developmental skills in their sleep.

In diverse American society culturally acquired and scientific knowledge of infant and childhood sleep often intertwine. Be that as it may, there are a few points on newborn and infant sleep that can help one to better understand their sleep needs. In the first three months, newborns seldom sleep for more than four-hour stretches without needing a feeding. Yet they usually sleep a total of fourteen to eighteen hours a day. From three to six months, you will observe newborn sleep maturity, a developmental process wherein most infants begin to settle down and are awake for longer periods during the day, some infants sleeping five-hour stretches at night. Therefore, between three to six months, you can expect your infant to have one or two nighttime awakenings. You will also see your infant's deep-sleep period lengthen. The vulnerable periods for awaking at night will decrease, and infants will begin to enter deep sleep more quickly.

Babies take longer to go to sleep, and they have twice as light sleep as do adults. Babies don't sleep as deeply as adults and have more frequent vulnerable periods for nighttime awakenings. Infants in the early months enter sleep through an initial period of light sleep. After twenty minutes or more, they gradually enter deep sleep, from which they are not so easily aroused. Some babies need help by being rocked or nursed to sleep. Infants have shorter sleep cycles than adults. Their cycles only last about fifty to sixty minutes. Babies therefore can be susceptible to waking as they cycle back to light sleep every hour or so. One of the goals of nighttime parenting should be to create a sleeping environment that helps the baby go through this vulnerable period without waking.

Dr. Joyce Walsleben, a sleep expert at New York University's School of Medicine, offers particularly good advice for parents of infants (A Women's Guide to Sleep, 2000). She suggests that parents organize their infants' sleep. Organization is built upon by encouraging the longest blocks of sleep at night, which means especially no stimulating play around sleep times. Parents should pick an awake-sleep schedule that works and is right for both Mom and her young infant and stick to it. Dad can also be included depending on the circumstances. Start by establishing a shared light-dark cycle within the home. The home should be dark at night, with just enough light to accomplish the necessary nighttime activities, and the light should be turned away from the baby. During the day the home should be bright, allowing for all necessary daytime activities, including indoor and outdoor play.

For years parents have shared what they called a neat method to help their young infants go back to sleep at night. Most parents did not know that what they were describing in its formal form was a technique called the Ferber method, developed by pediatrician Richard Ferber. This is a stepwise and progressive method for helping one's infant learn how to lull himself or herself to sleep. It also involves maintaining both daytime routines and night time rituals. Parent(s) put their baby down and then either leaves the room or returns to their own bed in the same room. Over the next several nights baby when he or she stirs or cries they are comforted or consoled at progressively longer intervals with baby eventually learning to sleep without crying or becoming upset. Pediatricians warn that this method does not work for all children especially for infants younger than six months and it may not appeal to all parents. Yet for many parents who are willing to try this method, it may lead to a satisfactory degree of success. One day I was in a popular coffee shop, and my waiter, a parent of a baby girl who had just turned two years old, told me that he uses the Ferber method and it works just perfectly; however, his wife, who cannot stand to hear their baby girl cry, has tremendous difficulty putting their baby down to sleep at night. I guess if nothing else, my waiter's story goes to show that at a very early age, children learn which parent they can manipulate and which one they cannot.

The Secret Language of Babies: The Five Cries of Newborns by Priscilla Dunstan is a DVD that contains five sets of cries of newborns that reflect five different basic infant needs. Dunstan is an Australian mother who claims she has a photographic memory for sound. At age four Priscilla was able to listen only once to an entire Mozart concert and then play it back precisely on the piano. She hears textures, colors, and resonance in a voice. She used these skills with her newborn son and began to see patterns in his cries. This newfound theoretical knowledge was used in researching the cries of over one thousand babies. During her eight years of research, five distinct cries were discovered that are universal. As a result of her research,

Dunstan claims that babies of different races and cultures all have the same distinct five cries. She further claims that since we all have the same reflexes, the sounds or cries that reflect these reflexes are the same. The five cries are similar, but if one listens carefully to the DVD, they can be distinguished. These five cries are only present in infants up to three months old and are most pronounced during a baby's pre-cry—before he or she starts crying hysterically.

A very interesting note is that cry #2, Owh, means "I'm sleepy"; it expresses tiredness. The "owh" sound is based on the yawning reflex. The first "owh" sound can be long and pronounced. The researchers found that the more tired babies became, the harder it was for them to fall asleep. Other signs of sleepiness include rubbing the eyes and yawning.

Perhaps this newly discovered universal baby language can help newborn infants sleep through the night and mothers to bond with their babies. Independent research of the Dunstan method in Sydney and Chicago, observing four hundred mothers, reported that 90 percent of the mothers found the system beneficial. Seventy percent reported their babies settled down faster, and 50 percent stated they felt a greater bond with their children.

More Postpartum Sleep Tips

- Lie down, rest, and put your feet up, even if you can't sleep. Don't use your desktop computer or laptop, talk on the telephone, or text-message unless it is really necessary.
- Enlist the help of others, such as your spouse or other responsible visitor in your home, in assisting you with nighttime feedings. Turning your infant's night feedings

over to someone else is easier if you're bottle-feeding, yet breastfeeding mothers still can take advantage of nighttime feeding assistance by introducing a bottle of breast milk early on so that someone else can provide relief in the middle of the night. Providing an extra bottle of pumped breast milk to be given by someone else can mean an extra two or three hours of sleep. Another alternative would be pumping at night to have the expressed milk on hand during the day for your help to provide while you nap.

- Help during the day can include older children who are able to take over household duties that you would normally perform. This will help prevent you from experiencing more fatigue than you already do.
- Nursing mothers can keep babies conveniently close to their bedside by placing a bassinet that attaches to the bed or sits next to it. Then they won't have to stir or move about their home as much to give nighttime feedings.
- Employ soothing sleep-inducing techniques when you have trouble sleeping.
- During the first several months postpartum, be discrete and use good judgment about when and how many guests to entertain in your home until you establish routines and schedules that work best for you and your family, including your newborn.
- Find time for stress-reducing activities during the postpartum time.

Sleep Tips for Menopausal Women

Fluctuating and decreasing levels of estrogen cause many of the symptoms of menopause. Many women in the perimenopausal and menopausal stages report sleeping problems. Many women often experience hot flashes, especially at night. Although total sleep time may not suffer, sleep quality often does. Hot flashes may interrupt sleep and cause frequent awakenings, leading to next-day fatigue, which in some cases can eventually lead to chronic insomnia. Other problems can include mood disorders, insomnia, and sleep-disordered breathing. These sleep problems are often accompanied by depression and anxiety.

Besides using low-dose estrogen replacement therapy, the use of soy products containing plant estrogens (called isoflavones) and other phytoestrogens can lessen the number and severity or prevent hot flashes. For many women (if not previously determined to be at increased risk for breast cancer), it may be worth a trial of phytoestrogens to try to curb or prevent hot flashes. Since estrogen enhances REM sleep, increases the time spent in REM sleep, and reduces the time it takes to get to REM sleep, this may be an added sleep-related benefit of taking phytoestrogens.

Other phytoestrogens include dong quai (angelica root), red clover, black cohosh, and ginseng. Dong quai helps the body use endogenous estrogens made from adipose tissue. Red clover contains isoflavones, which are chemically similar to estrogen. Black cohosh contains estrogen-like substances. Ginseng contains potent phytoestrogens and has been used for generations to relieve hot flashes. A concern in regard to dong quai is that it is contraindicated in women who have heavy bleeding in the perimenopausal period. There is some evidence that has implicated ginseng in abnormal uterine bleeding (endometrial hyperplasia) (Unfer, Casini, Costabile, Mignosa, Gerli and Di Renzo 2004) abnormal uterine bleeding (Albers, Hull, and Wesley 2004; Kabalak, Soyal, Urfalioglu, Saracoglu, and Gogus 2004). Ginseng at high doses (greater than 400 mg) can cause high blood pressure, gastrointestinal upset, and insomnia.

Other helpful sleep tips for women in menopause include:

- Eat healthy. Avoid large meals, especially before bedtime. If your taste allows, try eating foods rich in soy, as they may reduce the number or severity of hot flashes.
- Avoid foods that are spicy or acidic, as they may trigger hot flashes.
- Avoid nicotine, caffeine, and alcohol, especially before bedtime.
- Engage in regular exercise and maintain a regular, healthy weight.
- Dress in lightweight sleepwear to improve sleep efficiency. Avoid heavy, insulating bedcovers. In addition, one should consider using a fan or air-conditioning to cool the air and increase circulation.
- Effectively manage your stress, and as much as possible, avoid worrying. In an earlier section of this book about general tips for good sleep hygiene, there are a number of good strategies for handling stress, such as relaxation techniques, massage, and motion exercises such as tai chi or yoga.
- If you believe or someone you trust tells you that he or she thinks you are depressed, anxious, or having problems, don't be afraid to seek out the services of a mental or behavioral health professional to help you resolve your problems.

Sleep in Adult Men

Men's issues regarding sleep—while they often overlap with women's concerns—have unique aspects that the concerned male must understand. Men can have sleep-related conditions that affect them in certain ways. For example, men may experience different symptoms than women, and therefore some treatments and preventive strategies may affect men differently than women. In addition, in discussing sleep in adult men, one should probably take into account, at least to some degree, conventional established wisdom that men in general tend to care and know less about their health than women, men take more risks with their health, men tend to delay seeking medical help for their ill health, and men either deny or significantly play down their own weaknesses.

In 2004 Researchers at Pennsylvania State University College of Medicine asked twenty-five people, twelve men and thirteen women, to sleep in a laboratory for twelve consecutive nights. The first five nights, they were allowed to sleep for eight hours per night, and then for the next week, they were restricted to only six hours.

During the day the researchers performed computer tests of coordination on the subjects, measuring sleepiness and performance. They also measured hormones and cytokines, the latter being substances released by the body now well-known to cause inflammation. Both men and women scored approximately the same on the performance and daytime sleepiness tests. But the women adapted better to the shortened sleep time, using the time more effectively and enjoying more deep sleep than the men.

Men produce their entire daily complement of growth hormone during their sleep. In fact most of their GH production occurs during the early phase of sleep.Thus, the decrease in slow-wave sleep that men experience as they grow older parallels a related decline in growth hormone production in older men.

Daily testosterone levels fluctuate according to circadian and ultradian rhythms. The circadian rhythm (which represents testosterone's basal or tonic secretion) results in testosterone levels peaking during the mid-morning (around 8 a.m.) then falling during the mid-evening (around 8:00 p.m.) to its lowest level. The ultradian rhythm has an approximate cyclical oscillation of testosterone concentration every 90 minutes which is superimposed upon testosterone's ultraradian rhythm. Therefore, it is not so surprising, that testosterone levels are reduced by chronic sleep deprivation in males (Andersen, Alvarenga, Mazaro-Costa, Hachul, and Tufik 2011) and proper sleep is critical for testosterone regulation in men.

Sleep in Older Adults

The prevalence of insomnia is higher among older adults. According to the 2003 NSF Sleep in America Poll - Sleep and Aging, 44 percent of older persons experience one or more of the nighttime symptoms of insomnia at least a few nights per week or more. Insomnia may be chronic (lasting over one month) or acute (lasting a few days or weeks) and is oftentimes related to an underlying cause, such as a medical or psychiatric condition. Older people often obtain less amounts of sleep or don't feel as refreshed after a night's sleep because, as one ages, less time is spent in deep sleep, and thus, easy or early arousal may occur.

Unfortunately, as we age we tend to fall victim to more chronic disease. Disease affects sleep quality, and sleep quality affects the disease state. Much of the sleep disturbance among the elderly can be attributed to physical disease, psychiatric disorders, and the medications used to treat these conditions. Most age-related diseases will affect sleep and will be affected by sleep. For example, pain due to conditions such as arthritis or low back pain can affect how patients sleep, causing arousal during the night. Sleep-related breathing disorders can affect quality of sleep, result in sleep deprivation, and exacerbate medical conditions such as high blood pressure. In addition, these disorders tend to be more frequent in older adults. In certain disease processes, such as congestive heart failure, symptoms of shortness of breath can become worse during sleep. During the night while lying flat, patients may experience sudden episodes of shortness of breath, which disturbs sleep and contributes to daytime tiredness and fatigue, typical complaints characteristic of heart failure patients. To alleviate some of these problems, it is recommended that people with heart failure sleep with the head elevated.

Nocturnal sleep difficulties can result in excessive daytime sleepiness, attention and memory problems, depressed mood, physical decline, and lower quality of life. In addition, past research (Spira, Blackwell, Stone, Redline, Cauley, Ancoli-Israel, and Yaffe 2008; Yaffe, Laffan, Litwack Harrison, Redline, Spira, and Ensrud, et al. 2011) has shown that sleep-disordered breathing characterized by characterized by recurrent arousals from sleep and intermittent hypoxemia although common in older adults has a degree of association with dementia and cognitive deficits in the elderly. Older adults might have several other medical conditions for which they are seeking medical advice and treatment, yet they do not feel that they are getting any better. The result is that a tremendous amount of sleep disturbance and daytime sleepiness may go undetected and unrecognized. Conversely, the older adult may have a sleep disorder that might be complicating treatment of other medical conditions. As far as sleep disorders go, older women tend to experience more insomnia, while older men tend to experience more snoring, apnea, and other medical conditions that disrupt sleep.

In addition, there are physical changes that occur with aging. Specifically, there are sleep-pattern changes that are a part of normal aging, which often affect sleep quantity and quality. Studies on the sleep habits of older Americans show that as people age, many tend to have a harder time falling asleep (sleep latency), an overall decline in REM sleep, and an increase in sleep fragmentation (waking up during the night and for longer periods of time or having more difficulty staying asleep) than when they were younger. Older adults' sleep is shallower than that of young or midlife adults. This means there is less delta (or slow-wave) sleep, when growth hormone is produced. This latter sleep-pattern change is the classic sleep hallmark of aging. In summary, as we age, our sleep becomes less efficient (we tend to get less sleep for the time spent in bed).

Older people tend to become sleepier in the early evening and wake earlier in the morning compared to younger adults. This pattern is called advanced sleep-phase syndrome. The sleep rhythm is shifted forward so that seven or eight hours of sleep are still obtained, but individuals wake up extremely early because they have gone to sleep quite early. The reasons for these changes in sleep and circadian rhythms as we age are not clearly understood. Many researchers believe it may have to do with light exposure. Therefore, treatment options for advanced sleep-phase syndrome typically include bright-light therapy.

Luteinizing hormone released by the anterior pituitary gland binds to Leydig cells in the testes, stimulating the synthesis and secretion of testosterone. As opposed to healthy younger men, healthy older men do not achieve equivalent mean testosterone concentrations in a 24 hour period in response to pulsatile luteinizing hormone stimulation. Healthy young men regardless of whenever they sleep during the day demonstrate comparable blood testosterone levels during night time sleep, as long as they are able to sleep for the same duration (Axelsson, Ingre, Åkerstedt, & Holmbäck, 2005; Liu, Swerdloff, & Wang,

2005). As of the writing of this book there are studies under way which will help elucidate the bidirectional relationship between the sleep stages and release of testosterone. In addition, there are studies investigating the association between high or low levels of circulating testosterone levels and both known clinical sleep disorders and temporary sleep disturbances.

Of interesting note is that men, as they age, lose slow-wave sleep more than women (as a consequence there is less and less GH produced in men as they age and the GH pause in men occurs from about the age of 50 years onward into old age), but women report more sleep disturbances than men. In women the GH pause is brought on by the menopause.The prevalence of sleep disorders tends to increase with age. In fact, sleep apnea or restless legs syndrome appear with increasing frequency in older adults. The sum total of all these factors is that many older adults are reporting being less satisfied with their quality and quantity of sleep and feeling more tired during the day. However, a number of studies have shown that seniors who routinely exercise have fewer awakenings, fall asleep faster, and spend more time in deep sleep (Chen, Mei-Chuan, Liu, Huang, and Chiou 2012; Buman, Hekler, Bliwise, and King, 2011; Melancon, Dominique Lorrain, and Dionne 2015).

Older adults' sleep is shallower than that of young or midlife adults. This means there is less delta (or slow-wave) sleep, when growth hormone is produced. This latter sleep-pattern change is the classic sleep hallmark of aging. In summary, as we age, our sleep becomes less efficient (we tend to get less sleep for the time spent in bed).

CHAPTER 12

———◉———

Count Your Many Blessings, Not Sheep

Count your many blessings—not sheep. If you cannot sleep, do not stay up worrying about not sleeping—or anything else! Meditate on God's goodness and provision to you and those you love. Meditation is not a means to salvation or godliness, but a method of spiritual discipline, like prayer and fasting. The word "meditate" or "meditation" is mentioned twenty times in the Bible. For Christians meditation can be considered a form of worship, centered in love. Meditation is quiet focused reflection or contemplation before or after activities such as prayer, fasting, or reading Scripture.

What is the focus of Christian meditation? In a general sense, as we go about our day, we should follow the apostle Paul's guidance given in Philippians 4:8: "Finally, brethren, whatever things are true, whatever things are noble, whatever things are just, whatever things are pure, whatever things are lovely, whatever things are of good report, if there is any virtue and if there is anything praiseworthy—meditate on these things." It should also contain reflection on God Himself: His nature, His abilities, and His works.

In Joshua 1:8, God says to meditate on His Word day and night so we will obey it. The psalmist says this about the blessed man: "his delight is in the law of the Lord, and in His law he meditates day and night" (Ps. 1:2). As you fall asleep, meditate on Deuteronomy 33:27: "The eternal God is your refuge, and underneath are the everlasting arms."

Remember, Do Not Let the Sun Set ...

Under no circumstances go to bed angry, but strive at all times to be at peace with God, no matter what has happened to you. Because of life's many sorrows and disappointments, you may still awake during the night anxious or sad or the day's anger may stir in you again ... but immediately give it all on the altar of prayer to God, saying or even singing to yourself that it is well with your soul.

God knows your sorrow and your pain. His only Son, who was perfect and sinless, was crucified as a criminal. Jesus, who had been with Him since before the beginning of time, died a humiliating and cruel death, bearing all mankind's past, present, and future sin, shame, and evil in his body. It was in that moment of that perfect acceptable sacrifice that God turned away from Jesus because God did not want to look upon such evil sin and shame. Such pain, grief, and sorrow no other person can ever know. Yet because of His love for us, it pleased Him. Jesus was bruised for our transgressions; he was wounded for our iniquities and was raised to sit at the right hand of God, making intercession on our behalf.

When you are at your wit's end, pray and ask the Holy Spirit to intervene on your behalf. Let God know that you want His peace just for the night so that you can sleep and rest in Him. Do this every night if you have to until your storm is over.

"And the peace of God, which transcends all understanding, will guard your hearts and minds in Christ Jesus" (Phil. 4:7).

You can also ask others whom you know who love you and love God to offer intercessory prayer on your behalf. Because "the effective, fervent prayer of a righteous man avails much" (James 5:16 NKJV).

AFTERWORD

The Bible maintains the general view that sleep is necessary and good for mankind. Sleep is God's medicine, His good and perfect (in the sense of complete) therapeutic gift. Although we have made significant progress over many decades of studying sleep medicine and research, we still only have a notion of how blessed we are for this precious gift!

Our ability to be patient, long-suffering, loving, and forgiving is directly affected by the amount and quality of refreshing and rejuvenating sleep we receive.

"But the fruit of the Spirit is love, joy, peace, longsuffering, kindness, goodness, faithfulness, gentleness, self-control. Against such there is no law" (Gal. 5:22–23).

Proverbs 1:7 states, "The fear of God is the beginning of knowledge." It is through this reverential fear and awe of God that knowledge leads to true wisdom and understanding. God will honor scientists' work if they honor Him. Many Christian men and women have made some of the greatest scientific breakthroughs and discoveries in history.

Below is a list that may seem long, but it is only a partial list of great scientists who were devout men and women of faith seeking to understand God through His creation as well as the Bible.

- Nicholas Copernicus was the Polish astronomer who put forward the first mathematically based system of planets going around the sun.
- Sir Isaac Newton began his search for the laws of gravity and motion with this idea: God is a God of order; therefore, He must have laws that govern the universe.
- Johannes Kepler, mathematician and astronomer, discovered the formula for the orbit of planets around the sun. His works contained writings about how space and the heavenly bodies represent the Trinity.
- Robert Boyle, a famous chemist and one of the founders of the Royal Society, established Boyle's law for gases.
- Michael Faraday developed many of the laws of electromagnetism.
- James Clerk Maxwell invented color photography and discovered laws governing the distribution of molecules in gas.
- Lord Ernest Rutherford, a Nobel laureate in chemistry, has been called the father of nuclear physics.
- Joseph J. Thomson, another Nobel laureate, discovered the subatomic particle later named the electron.
- Louis Pasteur, the famous French chemist whom the world so honored by naming the sterilization process of pasteurization after him, also contributed to the development of the first vaccines.
- Joseph Lister, a British surgeon, defined germ theory and characterized the factors involved in wound sepsis.
- George Washington Carver, a pioneering agricultural chemist, botanist, and inventor, after the Civil War was credited with saving the South's financially devastated agricultural industry. He developed a crop rotation method to restore depleted soils from decades of growing only tobacco and cotton. He also invented over three hundred uses for the peanut and hundreds of other uses for soybeans, pecans, and sweet potatoes.

- Daniel Hale Williams performed the first successful open-heart surgery, and he was the first physician to open the chest cavity successfully without the patient dying of infection.
- Charles Richard Drew was a dedicated physician most noted for his research in blood plasma and for establishing the first blood bank.

It is interesting to note that on August 13, 1910, at the age of ninety-three, Florence Nightingale, the "mother of modern nursing" who completely reformed military medicine, died in her sleep. Throughout her life and career, "the lady with the lamp" maintained that her inspiration to do the work to which she committed her entire life was drawn from her "divine calling"; therefore, it is probably safe to say that God said to Florence Nightingale when she passed on to eternal life with Him, "Well done, my good and faithful servant. Come on in."

Despite the various significant contributions scientists have made to improve our understanding of life and our existence here on earth, they have yet to devise a means of prescribing a certain type of sleep as treatment for a specific medical or psychiatric diagnosis. It is my hope that after reading this book, you will realize a better understanding and appreciation of sleep as God's medicine. A holistic approach to proper sleep is important to actively maintaining our spiritual, psychological, and physical well-being—that needlessly elusive mind-body-spirit connection.

Finally, if you do not have a sleeping disorder, don't despair about the occasional difficulty sleeping—most people during their lifetime for one reason or another will have a few restless or sleepless nights. Often in these circumstances, one will be able to identify the cause and correct the problem on his or her own. It is only if difficulty sleeping persists or progresses over an extended period of time, that is, if it becomes chronic or recurrent, that one should seriously consider seeking professional advice. Start with your primary health-care provider, who will help you decide if you need further assistance from a sleep specialist. This professional can help you determine if you have a sleep disorder or not.

Even after having done all that you can, there is still no need to despair because just as Jesus reassured His disciples, He also reassures us through His Word: "These things I have spoken to you, that in Me you may have peace. In the world you will have tribulation; but be of good cheer, I have overcome the world" (John 16:33 NKJV).

The apostle Paul while in prison wrote to the church in Rome saying:

> And we know that all things work together for good to those who love God, to those who are the called according to His purpose. (Rom. 8:28 NKJV)

> Who shall separate us from the love of Christ? Shall tribulation, or distress, or persecution, or famine, or nakedness, or peril, or sword? ... Yet in all these things we are more than conquerors through Him who loved us. For I am persuaded that neither death nor life, nor angels nor principalities nor powers, nor things present nor things to come, nor height nor depth, nor any other created thing, shall be able to separate us from the love of God which is in Christ Jesus our Lord. (Rom. 8:35, 37–39 NKJV)

When I am feeling down for whatever reason and I am so troubled that I cannot sleep, I often meditate not only on passages and verses in God's written Word, but also on the many inspirational Christian songs that have been passed on to us throughout the years. Many years ago when I was a child growing up in Chicago, Illinois, my church pastor gave me the background of one of my favorite songs. It goes as follows: In 1873 Horatio Gates Spafford, a successful Chicago lawyer who had lost a great deal of his real estate investment in the great Chicago fire of 1871, was delayed by his business from accompanying his wife and four daughters (his son had died from scarlet fever around the same time as the fire) on a family vacation traveling by ship from New York to France. Therefore, he sent them on ahead of him. Off the coast of Newfoundland, the ship carrying his family collided with another ship and sank in high seas. Three of his four children were swept away by the sea waves. The mother, while holding onto a piece of driftwood, was able to hold onto the fourth child, but soon her strength and determination were overwhelmed by the sea and this child too was lost to the sea. The mother was eventually saved by the ship that struck them. She telegraphed her husband when she could nine days later: "Saved alone..."

Several weeks later Spafford was aboard ship crossing the Atlantic to be near his grieving wife. His ship passed near where his daughters had died. In his immeasurable grief and sadness, the Holy Spirit inspired him to pen one of the most beloved and inspirational hymns ever written. I have never forgotten this background of the hymn or the words to the hymn itself courtesy of the Library of Congress:

"It is Well with My Soul"

When peace like a river, attendeth my way,
When sorrows like sea billows roll;
Whatever my lot, Thou hast taught me to say,
It is well, it is well with my soul.

Though Satan should buffet, though trials should come,
Let this blest assurance control,
That Christ hath regarded my helpless estate,
And hath shed His own blood for my soul.

My sin—oh, the bliss of this glorious thought,
My sin, not in part, but the whole,
Is nailed to the cross, and I bear it no more.
Praise the Lord, praise the Lord, Oh my soul.

And Lord haste the day when our faith shall be sight
The clouds be rolled back as a scroll;
The trump shall resound, and the Lord shall descend,
A song in the night, Oh my soul! (Even so, it is well with my soul)

This book would not be complete without reiterating the greatest therapeutic gift of all—God's gift of love in Jesus Christ. In Him there is healing and respite for this sin-sick and desperate world. He is the Bread of Life, the living water, and the bright Morning Star.

APPENDIX A

Obtaining a Sleep Health History

Now that we have covered good sleep habits, sleep problems for the sexes, sleep patterns through the woman's life cycle, and CAT for the promotion of good healthy sleep, and furthermore, since we can all recognize that sleep is the choicest prescription ever written, how does one write God's sleep medicine prescription? I was taught many years ago that a good history beats a good physical any day. So let us start with a sleep health history (SHH). The history form provided in this appendix is one that any health-care provider can use; this means either the primary-care physician or specialist, the mental health specialist, the nutritionist, the chiropractor, the advanced-practice nurse, or other appropriate CAM provider. In addition, the lay reader of this book is invited to review the items listed on the SHH to become familiar with the type of questions on the form.

As with any prescription, it is necessary to use prudent judgment and always provide prescriptions judiciously. What am I saying here? Well, let us look at the practice of prescribing antibiotics. Overprescribing has led to widespread antibiotic resistance (strong and virulent bacteria survive, mutate, and come back even stronger and more resistant). Patients stopping their antibiotic medication before completing the full course as prescribed have also contributed to the increased incidence of antibiotic resistance and illness relapse. Under-prescribing has occasionally led to increased morbidity and mortality.

Because many individuals are ambivalent about change, especially if it involves significant changes in one's personal lifestyle and sleep habits, when taking a SHH, one should use the technique of motivational interviewing (MI) rather than lecturing or preaching during the process of information gathering.

Motivational interviewing involves careful listening, strategic questioning, and reflective listening in order to clarify and understand, and a nonjudgmental approach. This technique will help to ensure that the interviewer receives open, truthful, and honest communication and answers to the items on the history. One of the primary goals in this therapeutic interaction is to build a solid foundation for practitioner-patient communication and to engender a spirit of collaboration. This is vitally important in working together toward a healthier lifestyle and behavior change.

Motivational advice includes five components, best remembered by the mnemonic, "RAISE":

> *R*elationship with the patient
> *A*dvice to change
> "*I*" statements ("I am not going to pressure you to change")
> *S*upport for patient autonomy when making the decision
> *E*mpathy

At first glance conducting a sleep health history (appendix A) may appear to be a time-intensive endeavor, but one can gather this information over time and enlist other members of the health-care team to complete their portion of the history. In the long run, the time invested may actually shorten the time it takes to arrive at a diagnosis or treatment plan because of a higher likelihood of patient adherence.

SLEEP HEALTH HISTORY

Name_____ Gender_____M _____F Age____ (years)

I express gratitude for sleep through:	Always	Often	Sometimes	Rarely	Never
Prayer	_____	_____	_____	_____	_____
Meditation	_____	_____	_____	_____	_____
Blessings	_____	_____	_____	_____	_____
Heartfelt Thankfulness	_____	_____	_____	_____	_____

I plan and prepare for sleep by (Check all that apply):

Meditation _____

Warm Bath _____

Dimming the lights _____

Massage _____

Drinking a small glass of milk _____

Using Guided Imagery _____

Listening to relaxing music _____

Watching TV _____

Playing video or computer games _____

Talking on the telephone _____

Checking my e-mail _____

Reading a book _____

Practicing yoga _____

Practicing _____

Performing stretching exercises _____

Drinking a cup of regular coffee or tea _____

Drinking a glass of wine _____

Drinking a cup of herbal/non-caffeinated tea _____

Other _____ _____

Do you take recreational drugs? Yes_____ No _____

Do you drink coffee? Yes_____ No _____

Do you drink black tea? Yes_____ No _____

Do you smoke cigarettes? Yes_____ No _____

Do you drink alcohol? Yes_____ No _____

Do you sleep well (soundly)?   Yes_____   No _____

    If No, please state why here: _____

How many hours do you sleep at night during the weekdays?_____on the weekend?_____

In your opinion do you sleep too much?   Yes_____   No _____

              too little?   Yes_____   No _____

Do you feel sleep-deprived?   Yes_____   No _____

Do you experience daytime somnolence (falling asleep when it's important to stay awake)?

    Frequently (3+days/wk)_____Occasionally (3–5days/mo)_____Rarely (1/mo)_____Never_____

Do you experience daytime drowsiness?   Yes_____   No _____

    If yes, how often?   Frequently_____ Occasionally _____ Rarely _____

Do you nap during the day?   Yes_____   No _____

    If yes, how long?   _____15–30 mins   _____30–45 mins   _____>45 mins

Do you have problems breathing during sleep?   Yes_____   No_____

Do you snore?   Yes_____   No _____

Do you have sleep apnea?   Yes_____   No _____

Have you been diagnosed with a sleep disorder?   Yes_____   No _____

Do you get up at night to use the bathroom?   Yes_____   No _____

Are you taking medications to help you sleep?   Yes_____   No _____

If yes, please provide the name of the medication below (including over-the-counter drugs and nutritional supplements)

Medication Name	Dose	Frequency
_____	_____	_____
_____	_____	_____
_____	_____	_____
_____	_____	_____

	Alone	With one adult	With one child	With an adult & a child	With a pet
I sleep:	_____	_____	_____	_____	_____

161

Are you pregnant?   Yes_____   No _____

    If yes, how many weeks gestation are you? _____

    If no but you have given birth in the past year, how many months postpartum are you?_____

On most days my last meal of the day is at   _____a.m.   _____p.m.

	Small	Medium	Large
I consider this meal's size to be:	_____	_____	_____

Do you exercise?   Yes_____   No _____

    What form(s) of exercise do you participate in?_____

    When do you exercise (e.g., morning, afternoon, evening, night)?_____

    How many days out of the week do you exercise?_____

    How many minutes of exercise do you average during the week?_____

Is arguing before bedtime a routine in your household?   Yes _____   No_____

APPENDIX B

Keeping a Sleep Diary

A sleep diary (or log) usually includes daily times for:

- the time the person tried to fall asleep
- the time the person thinks he or she fell asleep
- the number, time, and length of any nighttime awakenings
- the time the person woke up
- the time the person got out of bed
- the time the person had wanted to wake up
- whether the person got up by himself or herself, by an alarm clock, or because of being disturbed
- a few words about how the person felt during the day
- the start and end times of any daytime naps
- what, if any, medications the person was using

A daily sleep diary expands on the notion of a sleep log and includes a chart with spaces for:

- the time you went to bed and woke up
- how long and well you slept
- when you were awake during the night
- how much caffeine or alcohol you consumed and when
- what/when you ate and drank

- what emotion or stress you had
- what drugs or medications you took

A sleep diary can help you discover:

- your natural sleep patterns or sleep-wakefulness cycles
- what time of the day that you are most alert
- what time of the day you function most efficiently
- how your lifestyle affects your sleep

SLEEP DIARY EXAMPLE

Name: _____   Sleep Diary Start Date: _____

Today's Date: _____

The time I went to bed last night: _____

After turning the lights off last night I fell asleep in _____ minutes.

I woke up today: _____ a.m. _____ p.m.

Specific number of times I awoke during the night: _____

If you experienced more than one awakening, the time (in minutes) for each awakening was:
1st awakening _____ 2nd awakening _____ 3rd awakening _____ 4th awakening _____

My sleep last night was interrupted for a total of _____ minutes.

After waking this morning I got out of bed at _____ a.m. _____ p.m.

Today, I took a nap at: _____ a.m./p.m. for _____ minutes
                        _____ a.m./p.m. for _____ minutes
                        _____ a.m./p.m. for _____ minutes

Last night I slept for a total of _____ (hours/minutes)

Overall quality of sleep (check all that apply): restful ___ refreshing ___ peaceful ___

Caffeine (cups)/time consumed	Alcohol (ounces)/time consumed	Food/other drink consumption/time consumed	Emotions/ stress at the time	Medication(s)/time taken
.	.	.	.	.
.	.	.	.	.
.	.	.	.	.
.	.	.	.	.
.	.	.	.	.
.	.	.	.	.

APPENDIX C

---⊙---

Glossary of Common Primary Sleep Disorders

All sleep disorders are comprised of a group of syndromes characterized by chronic disturbances in the quantity of sleep, quality or timing of sleep, or in behaviors or physiological conditions associated with sleep and interference in the ability to function normally. As of 2015 sleep experts have defined no less than 100 different types of sleep disorders. To qualify for the diagnosis of sleep disorder, the condition must be a persistent problem, cause an individual significant emotional distress, and interfere with personal, social, or occupational functioning. A primary sleep disorder is one that is not caused by an underlying medical or psychiatric condition, including drug or alcohol abuse.

Hypersomnia (hypersomnolence) is a condition characterized by excessive daytime sleepiness, prolonged drowsiness, excessive deep sleeping, or the inability to maintain wakefulness when desired. In terms of sleep duration, hypersomnia is defined as having sleep periods of ten hours or more at a time. Primary hypersomnia is most often seen in children. They have a normal variant sleep pattern with normal sleep efficiency, sleep/ wake cycles, and sleep architecture except they have longer sleep needs. This condition also may be a lifelong pattern.

Unfortunately, hypersomnia can also be a complication caused by both cancer and cancer treatments.

Primary Insomnia ("insomnia" is Latin for "no sleep") is the most common sleep disorder in adults. It involves a significant lack of high-quality sleep. It consists of difficulties in getting to sleep or staying asleep, waking up too early, or not feeling refreshed upon waking in the morning. It can be short-term or chronic. Insomnia may be caused by stress, anxiety, a change in time zones or sleep schedule, poor bedtime habits, an uncomfortable bed or bedding, or an underlying medical or psychiatric condition. Other symptoms include: difficulty falling asleep despite being tired; daytime drowsiness, fatigue, and irritability; the need for sleeping pills or alcohol to fall asleep; awakening frequently during the night, lying awake in the middle of the night, or awakening too early in the morning. In the acute form of insomnia, signs and symptoms last less than one or two months. Other forms of insomnia are: chronic, lasting greater than two months; and persistent insomnia, where signs and symptoms persist for twelve months or more despite treatment.

Jet Lag is a circadian-rhythm sleep disorder that occurs when a different time zone throws off the body's internal clock. It can take a few days to reset because sleep and wake patterns remain set to one's home time zone. It is characterized by disruptions arising from a mismatch between a person's circadian cycle and the cycle required by a different time zone. Frequent travel crossing many time zones makes one more susceptible to this type of sleep disorder. Working the night shift can mimic the symptoms of jet lag. Symptoms include: sleepiness during the *desired wake* portion of the day due to time zone change(s); difficulty sleeping during the *desired sleep* portion of the day; and difficulty altering one's sleep-wake schedule to one that is appropriate for the new time zone. There are other circadian-rhythm sleep disorders described in the clinical literature, the most noted being shift-work type.

A rule of thumb when traveling across the country: seek morning light when traveling west (travel as the sun rises, that, is east to west) and avoid morning light when traveling east (the red-eye to New York from Los Angeles is not a good idea if you have been awake all day). This guideline can help you reset your biological clock and avoid jet lag while traveling. In addition, make sure you get a few good nights' sleep before embarking on a trip that takes you across time zones.

Narcolepsy is a lifelong chronic neurological disorder that impairs the ability of the central nervous system to regulate sleep. It is mainly a disorder in adults, but it has been reported in children as young as three years old. Men and women are equally affected. Individuals experience extreme tiredness, with intermittent uncontrollable sleepiness, during the day, which can include involuntary napping. Narcolepsy is a dangerous sleep disorder because involuntary falling asleep can occur during activities such as walking, driving, or cooking, with drastic untoward effects.

Narcolepsy has three major symptoms in addition to sleep attacks: cataplexy, hallucinations, and sleep paralysis. Cataplexy involves sudden, short-lived loss of muscle control during emotional situations, with laughter being the most frequently involved emotion, followed by anger or excitement. It is thought that the condition involves a short interjection of REM sleep into a state of wakefulness. Hallucinations may occur just before falling asleep or right after waking up and are associated with an episode of REM sleep. REM sleep paralysis (lack of muscle movement except for eye movements, respiration, and the movement of the tiny bones in the middle ear) occurs during the transition from being asleep to waking up.

Nightmares or Night Terrors may be reactions to change, stress, or a frightening event. Sleep terrors often occur earlier in the night than nightmares and do not fully awaken the child. Unlike nightmares, sleep terrors lead to uncontrollable screaming, which may continue for some minutes even as you try to comfort your child.

Periodic Limb Movement Disorder (PLMD) involves muscle spasms of the legs (especially, the calves) or episodes of rhythmic jerking of the feet or legs during sleep, often to the point of disrupting sleep. This disorder is more common in the middle-aged and elderly. A mild form of PLMD is found at least in 45 percent of all older adults. It is more prominent in NREM stages 1 and 2 sleep. PLMD is frequently associated with RLS (Restless Leg Syndrome). According to the National Institute of Health's National Institute of Neurological Disorders and Stroke 80 percent of individuals with RLS also have PLMD. Many people with these disorders also report insomnia and daytime sleepiness.

REM Sleep Behavior Disorder—This condition occurs most often in middle-aged or older men. During REM sleep in response to dreaming, they engage in vigorous and bizarre physical activities, which are generally of a violent, intense nature. The sleeper tends to act out what's happening in his or her dreams, which could mean punching or kicking; thus, individuals with this disorder may injure themselves or their sleeping partners. This disorder is believed to be neurological in nature.

Restless Legs Syndrome (RLS) is a neurological movement disorder characterized by a cramp or some kind of irritation in the lower legs, which makes the person have an irresistible urge to move his or her legs or get up and walk around. In RLS, these unpleasant, tingling, creeping, or pulling feelings occur mostly in the legs, become worse in the evening and make it difficult to sleep through the night, and create discomfort and can compel the sufferer to move his or her legs, even while trying to fall asleep. Its prevalence increases with age, and about 10 percent of people in North America and Europe are reported to experience RLS symptoms. The cause of RLS is unknown, but it may be familial or a consequence of iron deficiency.

Obstructive Sleep Apnea (OSA) is caused by tissue collapsing in the back of the throat and blocking the airway as one attempts to inhale. OSA is characterized by brief but numerous involuntary breathing pauses (for ten seconds or more at a time) during sleep. These breathing pauses cause awakenings throughout the night, which allow for voluntary airway dilation. These awakenings make it next to impossible for sleep apnea sufferers to enjoy a night of deep, restorative sleep. Individuals experience gasping, gagging, or choking for air during sleep. Sleep apnea sufferers often feel sleepy during the day, and their concentration and daytime performance are impaired.

Sleep apnea affects between 2 and 10 percent of the US population. It is more common in men than in women and people who are middle-aged or older. While being overweight or obese are risk factors for sleep apnea, being thin does not preclude a diagnosis. This is a very serious disorder that can be life-threatening. Other forms of sleep apnea exist, such as central and mixed, but OSA is the most common form and reason for sleep laboratory referral.

There is an important clinical link between Type 2 diabetes and sleep apnea. In this group the severity of insulin resistance is correlated with the severity of sleep apnea. Specifically, past studies (Ip, B. Lam, Ng, W.T. Lam, Tsang, S. Lam 2002; Basoglu, F. Sarac, S. Sarac, Uluer, and Yilmaz 2011) have shown that sleep apnea is an independent risk factor for insulin resistance. In light of the many multisystem complications related to sleep apnea, it is incumbent upon all primary-care providers and their nursing staff to educate their diabetic patients in a nonthreatening, calm manner about the negative consequences associated with sleep apnea—especially if left untreated.

Sleep Starts—A common feeling of muscle jerks or a sensation of falling that happens when a person is just going off to sleep.

Sleep Talking (somniloquy)—Talking while you are asleep during NREM sleep. Vocalization is either in a few words (often mumbled) or a very short speech, most often in a low monotone voice. Usually this sleep disorder has no medical consequences unless incidents are accompanied by emotional outbursts or become frequent as to disrupt sleep. This disorder is mostly benign and is more common in children.

Sleepwalking (somnambulism) is partial arousal from sleep that occurs during NREM slow-wave stages 3 and 4 during the first part of the night. If an individual is awakened during a sleepwalking episode, he or she may be disoriented and have no memory of the behavior. In addition to walking around, individuals with sleepwalking disorder have been observed to carry out complex motor activities such as eating, using the bathroom, unlocking doors, or talking to others. Consequences can be dangerous, as falls and injuries have been known to occur. The disorder is most common in children eight to twelve years old. It is unusual for a primary episode of sleepwalking to occur in adulthood.

Sleep talking and sleepwalking occur in NREM sleep because the muscle paralysis that occurs in REM sleep precludes talking or walking.

Sleep or Night Terrors (*pavor nocturnus)* is a parasomnia in which a person awakes suddenly screaming or crying. Sleep terrors typically occur from partial arousal in stage 3 or stage 4 NREM sleep during the first third of the night. The individual has physical signs of arousal, like sweating or shaking, and generally is quite panicked. He or she may be confused or disoriented for several minutes, then fall asleep again and not remember the sleep terror episode nor recall the content of the dream the next morning. It is most common in children four to twelve years old and is outgrown in adolescence. In adults, it usually begins between the ages of twenty and thirty. In children, more males than females are affected with this disorder. In adults, men and women are equally affected.

APPENDIX D

Sleep-Related Terminology

Communal Sleep—"Cosleeping" or "bedsharing" (referring to bed in the generic sense of bedding down, whether on a bed, futon, mat, or whatever else is used) is sleeping with another person, usually a family member or friend.

Familial—A condition that tends to occur more often in family members than expected by chance alone.

Multiple Sleep Latency Test (MSLT)—Measures the onset of sleep by tracking the moment brain waves change from wakefulness to NREM stage 1 light sleep.

Sleep Debt is created when personal sleep requirements are not met. It is the difference between the number of hours one actually sleeps and the number of hours one should have slept. Sleep debt accumulates and increases quickly, but does not decrease spontaneously. The body reacts to a lack of sleep by having daytime drowsiness such that an intense desire to sleep induces the person to either go to sleep early or sleep in late.

Sleep Deprivation is not getting enough sleep or suffering disruptions to the sleep-wake cycle. It can occur over a period of months or even years before overt symptoms appear.

Sleep Fragmentation consists of periods of sleep that alternate with frequent awakening, resulting in that unrefreshed feeling upon final awakening to start the day.

Sleep Hygiene or *Good Sleep Habits* refers to the conditions and behavioral practices that promote and encourage routine, continuous, restful, and effective sleep.

Wakefulness—A state of awareness in which the individual is conscious of his or her surrounding environment and has the ability to interact with it. In the period before sleep, wakefulness is described as quiet wakefulness, where the individual is resting in a relaxed condition with his or her eyes closed.

Other Medical Terms

Dyspepsia—Difficult, disturbed, or painful digestion, which can lead to mild to severe gastrointestinal complaints or symptoms

Iatrogenic—Adverse state or condition consequential to the effect(s) of treatment by a physician, surgeon, or dentist.

Idiopathic—As relating to a medical condition or disease state, having an unknown or unclear cause.

Kegel Exercises—Pelvic floor muscle exercises practiced to help strengthen these muscles and to prevent urinary leakage.

Nosocomial—Acquired or caused by hospitalization.

Phytoestrogens—Plant-based compounds or chemicals with recognized estrogen-like physiological effects

Postpartum—Refers to the time period after childbirth.

RESOURCES

Sleep-Friendly Websites

www.sleepquest.com

www.thebettersleepcouncil.com

http://www.emedicinehealth.com/sleep_understanding_the_basics/article_em.htm

http://www.sleepeducation.com—Sleep education techniques

http://www.aasmnet.org—The American Academy of Sleep Medicine

www.sleepnet.com—Information on sleep disorders, with links to other sleep-related sites

http://www.asda.org—American Sleep Disorders Association

http://www.sleepfoundation.org—National Sleep Foundation, which supports sleep-related education, research, and advocacy

http://www.sleepeducation.org/healthysleep - National Healthy Sleep Awareness Project (2013-2018) sponsored by the Centers for Disease Control and Prevention

www.users.cloud9.net/*thorpy/—Information on clinical sleep medicine and research, government hyperlinks, sleep anatomy and physiology; also information for patients and consumers

www.sleepeducation.com—Sleep facts, sleep disorders, treatments and services; online interactive discussion forum

www-leland.stanford.edu/dement/children.html—Children and sleep disorders

www.apneanet.org—Apnea awareness, news, and education

www.americaninsomniaassociation.org—Insomnia, treatment options, support and resources, etc.

www.drowsydriver.org—The NSF's Drowsy Driver Education Program

www.healthtouch.com/level1/leaflets/sleep/sleep032.htm—Traveling and good sleep hygiene

www.rls.org – The Willis-Ekbom Disease Foundation (formerly the RLS Foundation)—Supports RLS research for cure and improved treatments of RLS, and increases awareness of this sleep disorder

Sleep Disorder Centers in the United States

A list of fully accredited sleep disorder centers can be obtained by contacting the American Academy of Sleep Medicine (AASM). Standards for accreditation are designed by sleep specialists, with a primary goal of ensuring that they reflect the latest advances in the diagnosis and treatment of sleep disorders. Treatment must include mechanical and pharmacological therapy. AASM centers must display and maintain proficiency in areas such as testing procedures and policies, patient safety and follow-up, and physician and staff training. Each center's minimal staffing must include a board-certified or board-eligible sleep specialist physician and certified sleep technologists.

Some centers are clinics, others are located within hospitals, others are freestanding laboratories only accredited as specialty laboratories for sleep-related breathing disorders, and a few are located in hotel inn settings. In fact, the inn-like setting is featured prominently in new center construction.

Many books and websites provide lists of accredited centers, but none of these lists designate which centers have insomnia programs or specialized insomnia services associated with them. Formal insomnia programs are continuing to grow in number. A small number of insomnia programs offer CAT. Some centers are still developing these programs and services. Other centers refer insomnia cases to medical psychotherapists. Still others maintain all their sleep-related services under the traditional umbrella of the sleep center. Some programs have a multidisciplinary team approach to treating insomnia that may include any combination of physician, psychologist, psychotherapist, acupuncturist, massage therapist, and other CAT providers. These services are provided on an individual or group basis or both. They sometimes offer support groups and patient education classes.

If you are interested in insomnia programs or services, please contact a sleep disorder or sleep medicine clinic or center in your local area for more information.

BIBLIOGRAPHY

Akestedt, Torbjorn. "Work Hours and Sleepiness," *Neurological Clinica* 25 (1995): 367.

Albers, Janet. R., Sharon K. Hull and Robert M. Wesley. "Abnormal uterine bleeding," *American Family Physician,* (2004), 69(8), 1915-1934.

American College Health Association – Healthy Campus 2020: Student Objectives. Available from http://www.acha.org/healthycampus/student-obj.cfm

Andersen, Monica L., Tathiana F. Alvarenga, Renata Mazaro-Costa, Helena C. Hachul, and Sergio Tufik. "The association of testosterone, sleep, and sexual function in men and women," *Brain Research* 1416 (2011): 80-104.

Argente, Jesus, N. Caballo, Vicente Barrios, M. Teresa Munoz, Jaime Pozo, Julie Chowen, and M. Lopez-Madrazo Hernandez. "Disturbances in the Growth Hormone-Insulin-Like Growth Factor Axis in Children and Adolescents with Different Eating Disorders," *Hormone Research* 48 supplement 4 (1997): 16–8.

Axelsson, John, Michael Ingre, Torbjörn Åkerstedt, and Ulf Holmbäck. 'Effects of acutely displaced sleep on testosterone," *Journal of Clinical Endocrinology & Metabolism* (2005), 90, no. 8, 4530–4535.

Ayas, Najib, David White, JoAnn Manson, Meir Stampfer, Frank Speizer, Atul Malhotra, and Frank Hu. "A Prospective Study of Sleep Duration and Coronary Heart Disease in Women," *Annals of Internal Medicine* 163, no. 2 (2003): 205–209.

Baillie, John. *Christian Devotion: The Theology of Sleep*, (London, England: Oxford University Press, 1962), Chap 11

Barger, Laura, Brian Cade, Najib Ayas, John Cronin, Bernard Rosner, Frank Speizer, and Charles Czeisler. Harvard Work Hours, Health, and Safety Group. "Extended Work Shifts and the Risk of Motor Vehicle Crashes Among Interns," *New England Journal of Medicine* 352, no. 2 (January 13, 2005): 125-134.

Basheer, Radhika, Robert Strecker, Mahesh Thakkar, and Robert McCarley. "Adenosine and Sleep-Wake Regulation," *Progressive Neurobiology* (2004), 73: 379–396.

Basoglu, Ozen K., Fulden Sarac, Sefa Sarac, Hatice Uluer, and Candeger Yilmaz. "Metabolic syndrome, insulin resistance, fibrinogen, homocysteine, leptin, and C-reactive protein in obese patients with obstructive sleep apnea syndrome." *Annals of Thoracic Medicine* 6, no. 3 (2011): 120.

Besedovsky, Luciana, Tanja Lange, and Jan Born. "Sleep and immune function," *Pflügers Archiv-European Journal of Physiology* 463, no. 1 (2012), 121-137.

Broussard Josianne, David Ehrmann, Eve Van Cauter, EsraTasali, and Matthew Brady. "Impaired Insulin Signaling in Human Adipocytes After Experimental Sleep Restriction: A Randomized, Crossover Study," *Annals of Internal Medicine* (2012), 157: 549-557.

Busch-Vishniac, Ilene J., James E. West, Colin Barnhill, Tyrone Hunter, Douglas Orellana, and Ram Chivukula. "Noise levels in Johns Hopkins Hospital,"

Journal of the Acoustic Society of America 118, no. 6 (December 2005): 3629-3645 doi: 10.1121/1.2118327.

Buman, Matthew P., Eric B. Hekler, Donald L. Bliwise, and Abby C. King. "Exercise effects on night-to-night fluctuations in self-rated sleep among older adults with sleep complaints," *Journal of Sleep Research* (2011) 20(1 part I): 28-37.

Buysse, Daniel, Barbara Barzansky, David Dinges, Eileen Hogan, Carl Hunt, Judith Owens, Mark Rosekind, et al. "Sleep, Fatigue, and Medical Training: Setting an Agenda for Optimal Learning and Patient Care," *Sleep* 26, no. 2 (March 15, 2003): 218–225.

Byberg, Stine, A-LS Hansen, Dirk Lund Christensen, Dorte Vistisen, Mette Aadahl, Allan Linneberg, and Daniel Rinse Witte. "Sleep duration and sleep quality are associated differently with alterations of glucose homeostasis," *Diabetic Medicine* 29, no. 9 (2012): 354-360. doi:10.1111/j.1464-5491.2012.03711.x

Cartwright, Rosalind, Alice Luten, Michael Young, Patricia Mercer, and Michael Bears. "Role of REM Sleep and Dream Affect in Overnight Mood Regulation: A Study of Normal Volunteers," *Psychiatry Research* 8, no. 1 (1998): 1–8.

Centers for Disease Prevention and Control Summary Health Statistics for U.S. Children: National Health Interview Survey (2002) Accessed May 12, 2006 at http://www.cdc.gov/nchs/data/series/sr_10/sr10_221.pdf

Centers for Disease Prevention and Control Summary Health Statistics for Adults: National Health Interview Survey (2002) Accessed May 12, 2006 at http://www.cdc.gov/nchs/data/series/ sr_10/sr10_222.pdf

Chen, Mei-Chuan, Hsueh-Erh Liu, Hsiao-Yun Huang, and Ai-Fu Chiou. "The effect of a simple traditional exercise programme (Baduanjin exercise) on sleep quality of older adults: A randomized controlled trial," *International Journal of Nursing Studies* 49, no.3 (2012): 265-273.

Davis, Scott, Dana Mirick, and Richard Stevens. "Night Shift Work, Light at Night, and Risk of Breast Cancer," *Journal of the National Cancer Institute* 93, no. 20 (October 17, 2001): 1557–1562.

Dement, William C. *Some Must Watch While Others Must Sleep.* (New York: W. W. Norton, 1978).

Dement, William C., and Christopher Vaughan. *The Promise of Sleep: A Pioneer in Sleep Medicine Explores the Vital Connection Between Health, Happiness, and a Good Night's Sleep.* (New York: Delacorte Press, 1999).

Dement, William C. "The study of human sleep: a historical perspective," *Thorax* (1998), 53 Supplement 3), S2-S7.

Dossey, Leslie. "Watchful Greeks and Lazy Romans: Disciplining Sleep in Late Antiquity." *Journal of Early Christian Studies* 21, no. 2 (2013): 209-239.

Djokanovic, Nada, Facundo Garcia-Bournissen, and Gideon Koren. "Medications for Restless Legs Syndrome in Pregnancy,"

Journal of Obstetrics and Gynaecology 30, No. 6 (June 2008): 505-507.

Dunstan, Priscilla. *The Secret Language of Babies: The Five Cries of Newborns* The Dunstan Baby Language DVD, 2006.

Earley, Christopher J. "Clinical Practice: Restless Legs Syndrome," *New England Journal of Medicine* 348, no. 21 (May 22, 2003): 2103–2109.

Ekirch, A. Roger, *At Day's Close: Night in Times Past* (New York: NY: W. W. Norton & Company, October 17, 2006), Part Two: Laws of Nature.

Engeda, Joseph, Briana Mezuk, Scott Ratliff, and Yi Ning. "Association between duration and quality of sleep and the risk of pre-diabetes: evidence from NHANES," *Diabetic Medicine 30* no.6, 2013: 676-680.

Environmental Protection Agency Report. Information on Levels of Environmental Noise Requisite to Protect Public Health and Welfare with an Adequate Margin of Safety. (1974). Available from http://www2.epa.gov/aboutepa/epa-identifies-noise-levels-affecting-health-and-welfare

Ferber, Richard. *Solve Your Child's Sleep Problems.* New, Revised Edition. (New York: Simon and Schuster, 2006).

Fiese, Barbara H. and R. D. Parke. "Introduction to the Special Section on Family Routines and Rituals," *Journal of Family Psychology* 16, no. 4 (2002): 379-380.

Fiese, Barbara H., Kimberley P. Foley and Mary Spagnola. "Routine and ritual elements in family mealtimes: Contexts for child well-being and family identity," *New directions for child & adolescent development*, 2006 (111): 67-89.

Flemons, W. Ward. "Clinical Practice: Obstructive Sleep Apnea," *New England Journal of Medicine* 347, no. 7 (August 15, 2002): 498–504.

Frank, Marcos G., Naoum P. Issa, and Michael P. Stryker. "Sleep enhances plasticity in the developing visual cortex," *Neuron* 30, (April 2001): 275-287.

Garbino, Sergio, Manolo Beelke, Giovanni Costa, Cristiano Violani, Fabio Lucidi, Franco Ferrillo, and Walter Swannita. "Brain Function and the Effects of Shift Work: Implications for Clinical Neuropharmacology," *Neuropsychobiology* 45, no. 1 (2002): 50-56.

Garcia, Jennifer. *Medscape Today, News.* "Hospital Noise Results in Significant Patient Sleep Loss" (2012). http://www.medscape.com/viewarticle/756575 (Accessed February 10, 2011).

Goodmote, Edward J. "Sleep Deprivation in the Hospitalized Patient," *Orthopedic Nursing* 4, no. 6 (November/December 1985): 33–35.

Gu, Fangyi, Jiali Han, Francine Laden, An Pan, Neil E. Caporaso, Meir J. Stampfer, Ichiro Kawachi, Kathryn M. Rexrode, Walter C. Willett, Susan E. Hankinson, Frank E. Speizer, and Eva S. Schernhammer. "Total and Cause-Specific Mortality of U.S.

Nurses Working Rotating Night Shifts, *"American Journal of Preventive Medicine* 48, no. 3 (2015): 241-252.

Hamada, A., J. Ishii, K. Doi, N. Hamada, C. Miyazaki, T. Hamada, Y. Ohwaki, M. Wada, & K. Nakashima. "Increased risk of exacerbating gastrointestinal disease among elderly patients following treatment with calcium channel blockers," *Journal of Clinical Pharmacy and Therapeutics* 33, no. 6 (2008): 619-624.

Harma, Mikko, and Juhani Ilmarinen. "Towards the 24-Hour Society—New Approaches for Aging Shift Workers?" *Scandinavian Journal of Work Environment Health* 25, no. 6 (December 1999): 610-615

Harinath, Kasiganesan, Anand Sawarup Malhotra, Karan Pal, Rajendra Prasad, Rajesh Kumar, Trilok Chand Kain, Lajpat Rai, and Ramesh Chand Sawhney. "Effects of Hatha yoga and Omkar meditation on cardiorespiratory performance, psychologic profile, and melatonin secretion," *Journal of Alternative and Complementary Medicine* 10, no. 2 (April 10, 2004): 261-268.

Hirshkowitz, Max, and Patricia B. Smith, *Sleep Disorders for Dummies.* (Hoboken, New Jersey: Wiley Publishing, 2004).

Hughes Jeff, and Judith Lockhart, Andrew Joyce. "Do calcium antagonists contribute to gastro-oesophageal reflux disease and concomitant noncardiac chest pain?" *British Journal of Clinical Pharmacology* [serial online] 64, no. 1 (July 2007):83-89.

Institute of Medicine Report. Crossing the Quality Chasm: A New Health System for the 21st Century. Washington, DC, National Academies Press, 2001.

Ip, Mary SM, Bing Lam, Matthew MT Ng, Wah Kit Lam, Kenneth WT Tsang, and Karen SL Lam. "Obstructive sleep apnea is independently associated with insulin resistance." *American Journal of Respiratory and Critical Care Medicine* 165, no. 5 (2002): 670-676.

Kabalak, Ayala A., Ozlem B. Soyal, Aykut Urfalioglu, Ferit Saracoglu, and Nermin Gogus Menometrorrhagia and tachyarrhythmia after using oral and topical ginseng. Journal of Women's Health. (2004), (7):830-833.

Kandil, Tharwat S., Amany A. Mousa, Ahmed A. El-Gendy, and Amr M. Abbas. "The potential therapeutic effect of melatonin in gastro-esophageal reflux disease." BMC gastroenterology 10, no. 1 (2010): 1-9.

Kawachi, Ichiro, Graham, A. Colditz, Meir J. Stampfer, Walter C. Willett, JoAnn E. Manson, Frank E. Speizer, and Charles H. Hennekens. 'Prospective study of shift work disease and risk of coronary artery disease in women," *Circulation* 92, no. 11 (1995): 3178-3182.

Knutsson, A. and H. Bøggild. "Shiftwork and Cardiovascular Disease: Review of Disease Mechanisms," *Reviews on Environmental Health* 15, no.4 (2000): 359–372.

LaBerge, Stephen and Lynne Levitan. Lucidity Dreaming FAQ 1.1 The Lucidity Institute, Inc. (Accessed March 15, 2007) at http://www.lucidity.com/LucidDreamingFAQ1.html#LD

Lanaj, Klodiana, Russell E. Johnson, and Christopher M. Barnes. "Beginning the workday yet already depleted? Consequences of late-night smartphone use and sleep," *Organizational Behavior and Human Decision Processes* 124, no.1 (May 2014):11-23

Lee, Kathryn A., Mary Ellen Zaffke, and Kathleen Baratte-Beebe. "Restless legs syndrome and sleep disturbance during pregnancy: the role of folate and iron," *Journal of Women's Health Gender-Based Medicine* 10, no. 4 (May 2001): 335-341.

Library of Congress Draft manuscript copy of hymn "It is Well With My Soul" by Horatio Gates Spafford created ca.1873-1878. Repository Manuscript Division, Source Collection: American Colony in Jerusalem, Digital Id http://hdl.loc.gov/loc.mss/mamcol.016

Liu, Peter Y., Ronald S. Swerdloff, and Christina Wang. "Relative testosterone deficiency in older men: clinical definition and presentation," *Endocrinology and Metabolism Clinics of North America* 34, no. 4 (2005): 957-972.

Manconi, Mauro, Vittorio Govoni, Alessandro De Vito, Nicolas Tiberio Economou, Edward Cesnik, Gioacchino Mollica, and Enrico Granieri. "Pregnancy as a risk factor for restless legs syndrome," *Sleep Medicine* 5, no. 3 (2004): 305-308.

Mander, Bryce A., Sangeetha Santhanam, Jared M. Saletin and Matthew P.Walker. "Wake Deterioration and Sleep Restoration of Human Learning," Correspondence *Current Biology* 21, no. 5 (March 8, 2011): R183-R184.
doi: http://dx.doi.org/10.1016/j.cub.2011.01.019

Marks, Gerald A., James P. Shaffery, Arie Oksenberg, Samuel G. Speciale, and Howard P. Roffwarg. "A functional role for REM sleep in brain maturation," *Behavioral Brain Research* 69, no.1-2 (1995): 1-11.

Marks, Gerald A., Howard P. Roffwarg, and James P. Shafferry. "Neuronal activity in the lateral geniculate nucleus associated with ponto-geniculo-occipital waves lacks lamina specificity," *Brain Research* 815 (1999): 21-28.

Martin, Paul. *Counting Sheep: The Science and Pleasures of Sleep and Dreams.* (New York: St. Martin's Press, 2002).

Massion, Ann O., Jane Teas, James R. Hebert, M. D.Wertheimer, and Jon Kabat-Zinn. "Meditation, melatonin and breast/prostate cancer: Hypothesis and Preliminary Data," *Medical Hypotheses* 44 (1995): 39-46.

Matthew P., Eric B. Hekler, Donald L. Bliwise, and Abby C. King: "Exercise effects on night-to-night fluctuations in self-rated sleep among older adults with sleep complaints," *Journal of Sleep Research* 20, (1 part I) (2011): 28-37.

Mayo Clinic™ Diseases and Conditions: Insomnia Basics - Risk Factors. Accessed June 18, 2013 at http://www.mayoclinic.org/diseases-conditions/insomnia/basics/risk-factors/con-20024293

McKenna, James J., and Lane Volpe. "Sleeping with Baby: An Internet Based-Sampling of Parental Experiences, Choices, Perceptions, and Interpretations in a Western Industrialized Context," *Infant and Child Development. Special issue: Parent-Child Cosleeping* 16, no. 4 (August 28, 2007): 359–385.

Melancon, Michel O., Dominique Lorrain, and Isabelle J. Dionne. "Sleep depth and continuity before and after chronic exercise in older men: Electrophysiological evidence," *Physiology & Behavior* 140 [serial online] (March 2015): 203-208.

Mindell, Jodi A., Lisa J. Meltzer, Mary A. Carskadon, and Ronald D. Chervin. "Developmental aspects of sleep hygiene:

findings from the 2004 National Sleep Foundation Sleep in America Poll." *Sleep Medicine* 10, no. 7 (2009): 771-779.

Moline, Margaret, Lauren Broch, and Rochelle Zak. "Current Treatment Options Links Sleep Problems across the Life Cycle in Women," *Neurology* 6, no. 4 (2004): 319–330.

Moore, Marcia, Stanton P. Nolan, Diem Nguyen, Samuel P. Robinson, Brenda Ryals, John Z. Imbrie and William Spotnitz. "Interventions to Reduce Decibel Levels on Patient Care Units," *American Surgeon*, 64 no. 9 (1998): 894-899.

Morris, Henry M. *Men of Science, Men of God: Great Scientists Who Believed the Bible.* (El Cajon, CA: Master Books, 1982).

Morselli, Lisa, Rachela Leproult, Marcella Balbo, and Karine Spiegel. "Role of sleep duration in the regulation of glucose metabolism and appetite," *Best Practice & Research Clinical Endocrinology & Metabolism.* 24, no. 5 (2010): 687-702.

Murphy, Gina, Anissa Bernardo, and Joanne Dalton. "Quiet At Night: Implementing a Nightingale Principle," *American Journal of Nursing* 113, no. 12 (December 2013): 43-51.

National Center on Sleep Disorders Research. Accessed May 12, 2006, at www.nhlbi.nih.gov/about/ncsdr/index.htm

National Highway Traffic Safety Administration, "Drowsy Driving and Automobile Crashes: Report and Recommendations, April 1998," Accessed May 12, 2006, at http://www.nhlbi.nih.gov/health/prof/sleep/drsy_drv.pdf.

National Institute of Health's National Institute of Neurological Disorders and Stroke – Restless Leg Syndrome Fact Sheet.

Accessed May 6, 2006 at http://www.ninds.nih.gov/disorders/ restless_legs/detail_restless_legs.htm

National Sleep Foundation. Sleep in America Polls: 2003-2012. Washington (DC): The Foundation. Available from: http://www. sleepfoundation.org/sleep-polls-data/

National Transportation Safety Board. Grounding of the U.S. Tankship Exxon Valdez on Bligh Reef, Prince William Sound near Valdez, Alaska on March 24, 1989. NTIS Report Number PB90-916405. Washington, D.C. 1990.

Neuendorf, Rache, Helané Wahbeh, Irina Chamine, Jun Yu, Kimberly Hutchison, and Barry S. Oken. "The Effects of Mind-Body Interventions on Sleep Quality: A Systematic Review," *Evidence-Based Complementary and Alternative Medicine* (2015): 1-17.

Nightingale, Florence. *Notes on Nursing: What It Is, and What It Is Not.* [First American Edition] (New York, NY: D. Appleton and Company, 1860): 44, 45-46.

Peguy, Charles. *The Portal of the Mystery of Hope.* Original translation published in the United States of America. Copyright © 1996 Wm. B. Eerdmans Publishing Co. 255 Jefferson Avenue S.E. Grand Rapids, Michigan 49503 All rights reserved. Authorized English translation of Le porche du mystère de la deuxième vertu. ©1929 by Gallimard, Paris. Critical edition, with preface and notes by Jean Bastaire. ©1986 by Gallimard, Paris.

Petrovsky, Nadine, Ulrich Ettinger, Antje Hill, Leonie Frenzel, Inga Meyhöfer, Michael Wagner, Jutta Backhaus, and Veena Kumari. "Sleep Deprivation Disrupts Prepulse Inhibition and

Induces Psychosis-Like Symptoms in Healthy Humans," *The Journal of Neuroscience* 27, no. 34, (July 2, 2014): 9134-9140.

PEW Research Center Internet and American Life Project Accessed December 20, 2014 at http://www.pewinternet.org/

Presidential Commission on the Space Shuttle Challenger Accident Report. Vol. 2. Appendix G. Human Factors Analysis. Washington, D.C. U.S. Government Printing Office; 1986.

Rafalson, Lisa, Richard Donahue, Saverio Stranges, Michael LaMonte, Jacek Dmochowski, Joan Dorn, and Trevisan M. Maurizio. "Short Sleep Duration Is Associated with Progression to Impaired Fasting Glucose: The Western New York Health Study," *Annals of Epidemiology* 20, no. 12 (2010): 883–889.

Richter, Joel E. "Gastroesophageal reflux disease. Severe Gastrointestinal Motor Disorders," *Best Practice & Research Clinical Gastroenterology* 21, no.4 (2007): 609-631.

Roehrs, Timothy and Thomas Roth. "Sleep, Sleepiness, and Alcohol Use," National Institute on Alcohol Abuse and Alcoholism. http://www.niaaa.nih.gov/publications/arh25-2/101-109.htm (Accessed Feb 14, 2013.)

Sadeh, Avi, Reut Gruber, and Amiram Raviv. "The Effects of Sleep Restriction and Extension on School-Age Children: What a Difference an Hour Makes," *Child Development* 74, no. 2 (2003): 444–455.

Schernhammer, Eva, Francine Laden, Frank Speizer, Walter Willett, David Hunter, Ichiro Kawachi, and Graham Colditz. "Rotating Night Shifts and Risk of Cancer," *Journal of the National Cancer Institute* 93, no. 20 (2001): 1563–1568.

James P. Shaffery, C.M. Sinton, Garth Bissette and Gerald A. Marks. "Rapid eye movement sleep deprivation modifies expression of long-term potentiation in visual cortex of immature rats," *Neuroscience* 110 (2002): 431-443.

Shilo, Lotan, Yaron Dagan, Y. Smorjik, Uzi Weinberg, Sara Dolev, B. Komptel, H. Balaum, and L. Shenkman. "Patients in the Intensive Care Unit Suffer from Severe Lack of Sleep Associated with Loss of Normal Melatonin Secretion Patter," *American Journal of the Medical Sciences* 317, no. 5 (May 1999): 278-281.

Sivertsen, Borge, Siri Omvik, Stale Pallesen, Bjørn Bjorvatn, Odd E. Havik, Gerd Kvale, Geir Høstmark Nielsen, and Inger Hilde Nordhus. "Cognitive Behavioral Therapy versus Zopiclone for Treatment of Chronic Primary Insomnia in Older Adults," *Journal of the American Medical Association* 295, no. 24 (2006): 2851–2858.

Spiegel, Karine, Esra Tasali, Plamen Penev, and Eve Van Cauter. "Brief Communication: Sleep Curtailment in Healthy Young Men Is Associated with Decreased Leptin Levels, Elevated Ghrelin Levels, and Increased Hunger and Appetite," *Annals of Internal Medicine* 141, no. 11 (2004): 846–850.

Spira, Adam P., Terri Blackwell, Katie L. Stone, Susan Redline, Jane A. Cauley, Sonia Ancoli-Israel, and Kristien Yaffe. "Sleep-Disordered Breathing and Cognition in Older Women," *Journal of the American Geriatrics Society* 56, no. 1 (2008): 45–50.

Stanchina, Michael, Muhanned Abu-Hijleh, Bilal Chaudhry, Carol Carlisle, and Richard Millman. "The Influence of White Noise on Sleep in Subjects Exposed to ICU Noise," *Sleep Medicine* 6, no. 5 (2005): 423–428.

Taheri, Shahrad, Lin Ling, Diane Austin, Terry Young, and Emmanuel Mignot. "Short Sleep Duration Is Associated with reduced Leptin, Elevated Ghrelin, And Increased Body Mass Index (BMI)," *Sleep, Abstract Supplement* 27 (2004): A146–A147.

The New King James Version of the Bible. New York: Thomas Nelson, 1982.

The Sleep Well. www.stanford.edu/~dement.

Tooley, Gregory A., Stuart M. Armstrong, Trevor, R. Norman, and Avni Sali. "Acute increases in night-time plasma melatonin levels following a period of meditation," Biological Psychology 53, no.1 (May 2000): 69-78.

Trotti, Lynn M., Srinivas Bhadriraju, and Lorne A. Becker. "Iron for restless legs syndrome," Cochrane Data Base Systematic Review 16, no. 5 (2012): CD007834.

Unfer, Vittorio, Maria L. Casini, Loredana Costabile, Marcella Mignosa, Sandro Gerli, and Gian C. Di Renzo. "Endometrial effects of long-term treatment with phytoestrogens a randomized, double-blind, placebo controlled study," *Fertility and Sterility* 82, no. 1 (2004): 145-148.

Van Dongen, Hans, Nicholas Price, Janet Mullington, Martin Szuba, Shiv Kapoor, and David Dinges. "Caffeine Eliminates Psychomotor Vigilance Deficits from Sleep Inertia," *Sleep* 24, no. 7 (2001): 813–819.

Vgontzas, Alexandros N., Emmanuel O. Zoumakis, Edward O. Bixler, Huong-Mo Lin, H. Follett, Anthony Kales, and George P. Chrousos. Adverse Effects of Modest Sleep Restriction on Sleepiness, Performance, and Inflammatory Cytokines. *The*

Journal of Clinical Endocrinology & Metabolism (2004), 89(5), 2119–216 1.

Wasleben, Joyce, and Rita Baron-Faust. *A Women's Guide to Sleep: Guaranteed Solutions for a Good Night's Rest.* (New York: Crown Publishers, 2000).

Webster, Gary. *The Wonders of Man: Mysteries That Point to God.* (New York: NY Sheed & Ward, 1957).

Webster's Universal Collegiate Dictionary Random House Value Publishing (2001) ISBN-13: 9780375425677

Wittern, Renate. "Sleep theories in the antiquity and in the Renaissance." *Sleep 88* (1989): 11-22.

World Health Organization - Guidelines for Community Noise (1999). *Guideline values 4.3.3 Hospitals.* Available at http:// www.who.int/docstore/peh/noise/Commnoise4.htm

Wyatt, James K. and Derk-Jan Dijk, Angela Ritz-De Cecco, Joseph M. Ronda, Charles A. Czeisler. "Sleep-Facilitating Effect of Exogenous Melatonin in Healthy Young Men and Women Is Circadian-Phase Dependent," *Sleep* 29, no.5 (2006): 609-618.

Yaffe, Kristine, Alison M. Laffan, Stephanie Litwack Harrison, Susan Redline, Adam P. Spira, Kristine E. Ensrud, Sonia Ancoli-Israel, and Katie L. Stone. "Sleep-Disordered Breathing, Hypoxia, and Risk of Mild Cognitive Impairment and Dementia in Older Women," *Journal of the American Medical Association* 306, no.6 (2011):613-619.

Yoder, Jordan. "Noise and sleep among medical inpatients: Far from a Quiet Night Sleep," Report *Archives of Internal Medicine (JAMA Internal Medicine)* 172, no.1 (2012): 68-70.

CPSIA information can be obtained
at www.ICGtesting.com
Printed in the USA
FSOW01n0540231216
28780FS